PAIN AND ITS ORIGINS, DIAGNOSIS AND TREATMENTS

UNRAVELING THE ENIGMA OF VISCERAL PAIN

VICTOR V. CHABAN, PHD, MSCR

NOVA BIOMEDICAL

New York

Library of Congress Cataloging-in-Publication Data

ISBN: 978-1-63483-430-8
Library of Congress Control Number: 2015951299

Published by Nova Science Publishers, Inc. † New York

Contents

Preface

The variations of symptoms and pain perception in a large percentage of patients diagnosed with various syndromes such as Irritable Bowel Syndrome (IBS), Painful Bladder Syndrome (PBS), Chronic Pelvic Pain (CPP) and others suggest the complex mechanism of etiology of visceral pain. Recent studies showed that modulation of visceral inputs of primary afferent nociceptors within lumbar-sacral dorsal root ganglia accounts for the observed changes in pain perception (nociception) and symptoms observed during the etiology of these syndromes. Patients diagnosed with these disorders frequently have pain from several organs. Moreover, for patients with IBS the most common co-morbid diagnoses include PBS or CPP. Even pain is strongly associated with the disease, the awareness to its pathology is further illustrated by the fact that the average time duration between the onset of pain and the diagnosis is 3 to 10 years. Viscero-somatic and viscero- viseral hyperalgesia and allodynia result in the spread of a perception of pain from an initial site to adjacent areas. Many patients may initially have only one pain source in the pelvis, but a multitude of mechanisms involving the peripheral and central nervous system can lead to the development of painful sensations from other adjacent organs resulting in pelvic pain. Pain research has uncovered important neuronal mechanisms that underlie clinically relevant painful states such as inflammation and neurodegeneration. The concept that the brain and other systems are closely connected in certain feeling states, especially in clinical presentations of chronic viscerally-associated nociceptive disorders, is widely accepted in scientific and clinical communities. Cells of the affected tissues may interact in cell-to-cell manner messages through the transfer of hormones, cytokines and prostaglandins that are released during pathological processes. Neurodegenerative diseases also accompanied by the concomitant decline in cognitive and motor performance therefore limiting normal body functions.

The complex interplay and balance between these diverse mediators, ageing, genetic background, and environmental factors may ultimately determine the outcome of the progression of chronic visceral pain. On a molecular level, these responses are highly complex, involving a vast array of messenger molecules interacting with enzymes and receptors of virtually every class, directing recruitment of many types of cells to recover the healthy state. Indeed, a balance between the messengers with the inherent redundancy of the different body systems makes therapeutic intervention a considerable challenge.

Taking into the consideration a rapid growth of scientific knowledge the impact on society of a successful translation of a basic or clinical observation into new therapies is substantial. Today, understanding and meeting public concerns are as important as performing clinical studies. Despite many advances, the pathophysiological mechanism of visceral pain is still poorly understood comparing with its somatic counterpart and, as a result, the therapeutic efficacy is usually unsatisfactory. Even after tissue healing, pain may persist as chronic pain with a major impact on quality of life. To date, the majority of publications on chronic pain adopt an empirical approach to the treatment of visceral pain, primarily based on dealing with the putative nociceptive source of the pain. Most of the current data pertains to specific functional syndromes defined by medical subspecialties: IBS (gastroenterology); chronic pelvic pain: CPP (gynecology); interstitial cystitis/painful bladder syndrome: IC/PBS (urology); fibromyalgia (rheumatology) and others. Many reports describe the substantial overlaps between two or more of these syndromes. Moreover, clinical presentations of functional syndromes lack a specific pathology in the affected organ but may respond to a viscero-visceral cross-sensitization in which increased nociceptive input from an inflamed organ (i.e., uterus) sensitizes neurons that receive convergent input from an unaffected organ (i.e., colon or bladder) however the site of visceral cross-sensitivity is unknown. In this book, the author aims to challenge the traditional concept of many painful syndromes among different medical sub-disciplines for which therapies are developed by distinct divisions within pharmaceutical sciences to provide a systematic mechanism-orientated approach to the etiology of visceral pain and to present potential new therapies for various pain-associated disorders.

This book represents an attempt to review the most recent knowledge concerning nociceptive processes occurring in the visceral organs. At present, the available information concerning the regulation of nociception have been dramatically multiplied. Paradoxically, proposed therapeutic intervention is sometimes complicated by new data. Some of these data, even being correct, are contradictory due to different models and methodological approaches used for their collection. I hope this book can help health care providers, researchers and students in various disciplines of medicine or basic sciences to increase their knowledge concerning all aspects of visceral pain, as well as look for new concepts and approaches in this important topic. Reaching further than the concrete basic science contribution, this project is a liaison between the basic science work and the clinical aspects that are addressed through other disciplines such as anesthesiology (pain management), gastroenterology, urology and gynecology. Over the last decade, medical literature has carefully documented the undertreatment of all types of pain by physicians especially in vulnerable populations in medically underserved areas that receive almost no attention from the medical community. From a public health prospective, a substantial impact on our knowledge of nociceptive diseases can help to achieve a better quality of life for patients affected by visceral pain, leading to the discovery of new therapeutic interventions.

Victor V. Chaban, PhD, MSCR
Charles R. Drew University of Medicine and Science
University of California, Los Angeles, USA
Email: chaban@ucla.edu

Introduction

The concept of the brain's close connection to pelvic viscera plays an important role in certain feeling states especially in clinical presentations of chronic viscerally-associated nociceptive disorders. This concept is now widely accepted in scientific and clinical communities. Moreover, the fact that primary afferent neurons modulate nociception supports the idea about the involvement of the peripheral central system in the etiology of a wide range of functional and inflammatory gastrointestinal diseases that may potentially lead to new interventions and therapies.

Chest pain from coronary heart disease, endometriosis, acute and recurrent/chronic pelvic pain or abdominal pain from irritable bowel syndrome are all visceral pain sensations that may result in part from sensitization or sensory neurons. As we begin the investigation of particular problems that underlie visceral pain in the central nervous system (CNS) and peripheral nervous system (PNS), it may be asked - just what is so special about primary afferents? These nerve cells have two special properties that distinguish them from all other cells in the body. First, they conduct an input from the internal or external environment for long distances without any loss of signal strength. Second, they possess an intercellular connection within the ganglia or with other neurons that determine the type of information (sensation) and range of responses they can yield toward the CNS. Sensitization of primary afferent neurons to stimulation may play a role in the enhanced perception of visceral sensation and pain. Mechanisms of peripheral sensitization may involve increased transduction, which is secondary to repeated stimulation or an increase in the excitability of the afferent nerves by molecules that decrease the excitation threshold. Sensitization can also develop in response to inflammation although basic mechanisms of this process are poorly understood.

Pain is a protective mechanisms that alerts the individual to a condition or experience that is harmful to the body. Somatic pain is superficial and originates from the areas close to the surface of the body. Visceral pain originates in internal organs, the abdomen or the skeleton. The accumulation of disabilities and nociceptive diseases that limit normal body functions is a major risk factor for the quality of life. Many nociceptive diseases accompanied by the concomitant decline in cognitive and motor performance share the same pathophysiological changes. Pain is one of the body's most important adaptive mechanisms, and all current definitions suggest it is a complex phenomenon that cannot solely be explained as a response to injury. Different systems interact to produce pain sensation. The sensory system processes information regarding the strength, intensity, and temporal/spatial aspects of nociception. The affective system determines the individual's conditioned avoidance behavior. The evaluative system overlies the individual's learned experience of pain. The afferent pathways which begin in the PNS at the level of dorsal root ganglion (DRG) send information to the spinal gate in the dorsal horn and then ascend into the CNS centers. The sensory process leading to the perception of pain is called nociception. Nociceptors are free nerve endings that respond to thermal, mechanical or chemical stimuli. Because they are not distributed evenly in the body, the sensitivity to pain differs according to the body area. Some of the triggering mechanisms of nociception initiate release of neuromodulators and lymphokines, and chronic inflammatory mediators. Most common excitatory (pro-nociceptive) neuromodulators include substance P, glutamate, somatostatin, VIP (vasoactive intestinal peptide), CGRP (calcitonin-gene-related peptide) and ATP (adenosine- triphosphate). Most common inhibitory (anti-nociceptive) neuromodulators include GABA (γ-aminobutyric acid), glycine, serotonin, norepinephrine and endorphins. Endorphins (endogenous morphines) inhibit transmission of pain by binding to mu, delta and kappa opioid receptors. Cells of the affected tissues may interact in a cell-to-cell manner messages through the transfer of hormones, cytokines, and autacoids such as histamine, serotonin, kinins and prostaglandins released in pathological processes. The complex interplay and balance between these diverse mediators, ageing, genetic background, and environmental factors may ultimately determine the outcome of progression of neurodegeneration, one of a major clinical problem associated with nociception. On a molecular level, these responses are highly complex, involving a vast array of messenger molecules in addition to neuromodulators interacting with enzymes and receptors of virtually every class, directing the recruitment of many types of cells to recover the healthy state of individual. Indeed, a balance between the messengers with the inherent redundancy of the different body systems makes therapeutic intervention a considerable challenge.

The present book is written at the basis of available publications and several authors' recent reviews (Chaban 2012-2015) and my research experience in this field. It also includes novel ideas, not previously published. Data are summarized in separate chapters with references to corresponding manuscripts and reviews. The text gives a lucid view of novel aspects of pain generation and perception. It is recommended to students, scientists, health care providers and patients who seek a fundamental understanding of neuronal modulatory systems. This book is not intended to be a comprehensive review of all currently known regulatory mechanisms associated with nociception, but rather aims to provide a framework for understanding the most significant signaling processing in order to unravel the enigma of visceral pain.

References

Chaban V. Estrogen and Visceral Nociception at the Level of Primary Sensory Neurons. *Pain Research and Treatment*, Volume 1, 2012.

Chaban V. Primary Afferent Nociceptors and Visceral Pain, In "Endometriosis - *Basic Concepts and Current Research Trends*," In Tech, 2012, p. 367-381.

Chaban V. Role of primary afferent nociceptors in visceral pain associated with Irritable Bowel Syndrome. In: "*Irritable Bowel Syndrome: Symptoms, Diagnosis and Treatment Options*," NOVA Publishers, 2012.

Chaban V. Estrogen Preferentially Acts on Visceral Afferents to Modulate the Nociception, *Journal of Autacoids*, 2013, 2:1.

Chaban V. Estrogen Modulation of Visceral Nociceptors. *Current Trends in Neurology* 2013, 7, p. 51- 55.

Chaban V. Chronic Pelvic Pain: Focus on Etiology and Modulation, *International Journal of Research in Nursing*, 2014, 5 (1): 1-2.

Chaban V. Visceral Pain: Basic Research Concepts and Therapeutic Interventions, *International Journal of Research in Nursing*, DOI: 10.3844/ijrn.2015.

Chapter 1

Pathways of Nociception

Abstract

This chapter provides basic knowledge concerning different mechanisms of pain transmission- nociception. The pain field has been advocating for some time for the importance of teaching people how to live well with pain and we might again consider the possibility that we can help people live well without pain. This refers to a range of educational interventions that aim to change one's understanding of the biological mechanisms associated with nociception. Pain is a hallmark of almost all bodily ailments and can be modulated by agents, including analgesics and anesthetics that suppress pain signals in the nervous system. Defects in the modulatory systems, including the endogenous pain-inhibitory or pain- excitatory pathways, are a major factor in the initiation and chronicity of pain. The Gate Control Theory is presented with discussion on the capacity of pain modulation to cause both hyper- and hypoalgesia. An emphasis has been given to highlight receptors and their ligands involved in visceral pain.

Etiology of Pain

International Association for the Study of Pain defines pain as "unpleasant sensory and emotional experience associated with actual or potential tissue damage or described in terms of such damage." McCaffery (1980) defined pain as "whatever the experiencing person says it is, existing whenever he says it does." Pains that are evoked by noxious sensory inputs have been meticulously investigated by scientists, and their signal transduction mechanisms are generally well understood. In contrast, visceral pain syndromes, which are often characterized by severe pain associated with little or no discernible injury or pathology, remain a mystery. Unrelieved pain has major negative effects on the lives of millions of people worldwide, and is associated with huge societal costs. Breakthroughs in pain therapy have been rare in the past 50 years, but there is increasing hope that advances in multiple areas of pain research could lead to the introduction of much-needed novel and more effective analgesics (Melzak 2008).

The specificity theory of pain was described by Descartes in the seventeenth century and proposes that the intensity of pain is directly related to the amount of associated tissue injury. Later, specificity theory proposes that a mosaic of specific pain receptors in body tissue projects to a pain centers in the brain. It is useful to explain acute pain but does not account for chronic or cognitive and psychological contributions to nociception. The traditional theory of pain, which evolved during the twentieth century, states that pain is a specific sensation produced by a direct-line pain pathway from pain receptors in the body to a pain center in the brain. The gate control theory of pain, proposed in 1965 by Melzak and Wall, focused on chronic pain and postulated that neural gates in the spinal cord can be opened or closed by signals descending from the brain, as well as by sensory information ascending from the body. This theory also highlighted the psychological functions of the brain and produced an explosive growth of knowledge related to pain. Brain research, especially in neuropharmacology and cognitive neuroscience, has led to the development of new drugs, as well as several psychological techniques that produce substantial relief from chronic pain. The gate control theory also stimulated a shift away from the traditional direct-line pain pathway to the concept of parallel neural networks in the brain associated with the sensory, affective and cognitive dimensions of pain (Melzak 2005). New approaches to reveal the nociceptive functions of the brain will hopefully lead to the relief of the pain and suffering that is currently endured by millions of people.

Visceral pain is the most common form of pain caused by varied diseases and a major reason for patients to seek medical consultation. Despite decades of extensive research and the availability of several therapeutic options, management of patients with chronic visceral pain is often inadequate, resulting in frustration for both patients and physicians. This is, most likely, because the mechanisms associated with chronic visceral pain are different from those of acute pain. For years, treatment recommendations for visceral pain were the same as that for somatic pain. However, it is widely accepted that visceral pain processing is distinctly different from somatic pain and as a result it should be treated differently (Kannampalli and Sengupta 2015). It also known that the pathophysiology of the visceral pain is extremely complex. The gate control theory's most important contribution to biological and medical science was its emphasis on central nervous system (CNS) mechanisms. In this book the author will present new scientific evidence of regulation of visceral pain in peripheral nervous system (PNS) at the level of primary afferent neurons located in dorsal root ganglia (DRG). DRG neurons have very characteristic cytoplasmic organelles regardless of their size. Neuronal cytoplasm in the perikaryon is reach in smooth and rough endoplasmic reticulum connoting an emphasis on their secretory activity. These neurons are rich in mitochondria, connoting their dependence on high rates of adenosine-triphosphate (ATP) generation. Neuronal processes (neuritis) exhibit prominent microtubules to maintain their polarized shapes.

Primary order neurons: nociceptors bare nerve endings in skin, muscle, joints, arteries, and the viscera that respond to chemical, mechanical, and thermal stimuli. They can detect a wide range of stimuli through A-delta fibers or unmyelinated C polymodal fibers. These neurons communicate to second and third order neurons in spinal cord and primary somatosensory cortex providing segmental regulation of nociception. Neuromodulation of pain provides diffuse noxious control and integration of peripheral sensory axon terminals, spinal interneurons by top-down control pathways. PNS stimuli converge on the spinal dorsal horns. Additionally, threshold depolarization from inflammatory mediators after nociception leading to hyperalgesia and allodynia. Historically, it was believed nervous system fails to mount an inflammatory response due to its protection from the systemic immune system mediated by blood-brain barrier. However, in the last decades it became more evident role of inflammatory response induced within CNS and PNS. Various cytokines possess a significant role in nerve pathology and their presence is fundamental for the repair, regeneration and neurological recovery. The most interesting aspect of this recovery is the new concept that the concentration of cytokine seems to be criteria for determining their function and possible physiological response, Progress has been made in understanding the mechanisms underlying the action of cytokines in pain. To date, several direct and indirect pathways are known that link cytokines with nociception or hyperalgesia. Cytokines may act via specific cytokine receptors inducing downstream signal transduction cascades, which then modulate the function of other receptors like the ionotropic glutamate receptor, the transient vanilloid receptors, or sodium channels. This receptor activation, either through amplification of the inflammatory reaction, or through direct modulation of ion channel currents, then results in pain sensation. Complete understanding of the basis for nociceptive signal transduction initiated by primary afferent neurons requires knowledge of all the molecules involved. Before we can deal with the critical details of molecules that regulate the function of DRG neurons, we must consider how these cells are differ from the other cells in the body. They are excitable and capable of communication. Contrary to what one might assume, the more we learn about intercellular communication within DRG, the more complicated the situation appears. Many chemicals and neurotransmitters involved in this neuromodulation: pain excitatory (glutamate, aspartate) or pain inhibitory (serotonin, GABA, endorphins). Evidence from extensive clinical and basic research in the last decade have shown the involvement of several receptors and ion channels in the development and maintenance of chronic visceral pain conditions (Table 1.1). On the basis of their functional actions, amino acid neurotransmitters have been divided into two categories: excitatory (glutamate, aspartate) which depolarize neurons and inhibitory (γ- aminobutyric acid: GABA, gycine, taurine) which hyperpolarize neurons. Among them are GABA, the major inhibitory transmitter and glutamate, the major excitatory in the brain, and glycine, important inhibitory transmitter in the brain stem and spinal cord. GABA produces neuronal inhibition by acting on a diversity of membrane-bound receptors. These receptors can be divided into two major types: ionotropic receptors that are ligand-gated ion channels (GABA-a receptors), and metabotropic receptors that are G-protein coupled receptors (GABA-b receptors).

The excitatory amino acid, glutamate, is a major neurotransmitter in the CNS and plays an important role in nociceptive processing via a diverse set of membrane receptors which include both ionotropic and metabotropic. Activation of these receptors is responsible for basal excitatory synaptic transmission and many forms of synaptic plasticity such as long-term potentiation (LTP) and long-term depression. Glutamate acts on three ionotropic receptor subtypes: N-methyl-D-aspartate receptor (NMDA), α-amino-3-hydroxy-5-methyl-4-isoxazolepropionic acid receptor (AMPA), and kainite receptors that are widely reported to be involved in plasticity, brain development, learning, excitatory synaptic transmission, and LTP. NMDA receptors are calcium channels activated by glutamate and are slowly desensitized once activated. These high-calcium permeable channels generate synaptic neuroplasticity, wide dynamic range neuronal responses and gene expression.

Table 1.1. List of Receptors Involved in Visceral Nociception and Their Ligands

Receptor		Agonist	Antagonist
P2X3		ATP, αβ-met ATP	AF 219
GABA A receptor		GABA, Muscimol, HZ166	Baclofen
GABA B receptor		GABA, Baclofen, gamma-hydroxybutyrate, CGP7930	Phaclofen, CGP-35348
NMDA receptor		NMDA, glutamate, aspartic acid	AP-5, AP-7, Ketamine
Kainate receptor		Kainic acid	LY382884, CNQX, DNQX
AMPA receptor		AMPA, glutamate	NBQX, Kynurenic acid
Opioid receptor			
MOR		Morphine, oxycodone	-
KOR		Oxycodone, asimadoline	-
DOR		Enkephalin, cannabidiol, tetrahydrocannabinol	Buprenorphine
Cannabinoid (CB) receptor	CB1	Dronabinol	-
	CB2		
Serotonin (5-HT) receptor	$5\text{-}HT_1$	DPAT	-
	$5\text{-}HT_3$	-	Alosetron
	$5\text{-}HT_4$	Tegaserod	-
TRP channels	TRPV1	-	SB 366791
	TRPA1	-	-
	TRPV4	-	RN1734
	TRPC4	-	ML-204

ATP, adenosine-tri-phosphate; GABA, gamma aminobutyric acid; NMDA, N-methyl-D-aspartate receptor; AMPA, α-amino-3-hydroxy-5-methyl-4-isoxazolepropionic acid receptor; MOR, μ-opioid receptor; KOR, κ-opioid receptor; DOR, δ-opioid receptor; DPAT, 8-hydroxy-DPAT hydrobromide; TRP, transient receptor potential.

Our previous data showed involvement of NMDA (Chaban et al. 2004) and group II metabotropic glutamate receptors (Chaban et al. 2011) in modulation of nociception in PNS by modulating DRG neuronal activity. In addition, NMDA receptors appear to have a pivotal role in long-term depression (LTD), long-term potentiation (LTP), and developmental plasticity. However, overactivation or prolonged stimulation of NMDA receptors can damage and eventually kill neurons via process called excitotoxicity. AMPA and kainic acid (KA) receptors mediate fast excitatory synaptic transmission and are associated primarily with voltage-independent channels that gate a depolarizing current carried by the influx of sodium ions.

Opioid receptors are a group of G protein-coupled receptors with opioids as ligands. Kappa and mu opioid receptors are found on visceral afferents. Moreover, kappa opioid receptor expression is functionally up-regulated during inflammation and chronic visceral hypersensitivity. The cannabinoid (CB) receptors in mammals are CB1 and CB2, both members of the superfamily of G protein-coupled receptors. CB1 receptors are found primarily in neurons of the brain and GI tract extrinsic and intrinsic nervous system while CB2 receptor is expressed mainly in the immune system. Both receptors are G-protein- coupled. The role of CB receptors in visceral pain is unclear and their role in modulation of nociception is a subject of intense research. The transient receptor potential (TRP) family of ion channels is TRPV1, TRPV2, TRPV3, TRPV4, TRPM 8, and TRPA1. These channels are, in general, thermoreceptors found on poorly myelinated and nonmyelinated afferents arising from CNS and PNS (dorsal root and nodose ganglia). TRPA1 is highly expressed on primary afferents. Another potential target receptor in regulating nociception is purinergic P2X3 receptors (Burnstock 2013). Over the last decade author of this book was involved in research studies that confirmed that both TRPV1and purinoregic- mediated mechanosensory transduction are involved in the initiation of visceral pain (Chaban et al. 2003; Chaban 2008; Cho and Chaban 2012a; Cho and Chaban 2012b). I believe the great challenge ahead of us is to further explore the role of known and discover new signal transduction pathways of visceral pain.

References

Burnstock G. Purinergic signalling: pathophysiology and therapeutic potential. *Keio J Med*. 2013; 62(3): 63-73.

Chaban V., Mayer E., Ennes H., Micevych P. Estradiol inhibits ATP-induced $[Ca^{2+}]_i$ increase in DRG neurons *Neuroscience* 2003, 118 (6), 941-948.

Chaban V., Li, J., Ennes H., Nie J., Mayer E., McRoberts J. N-methyl D-aspartate (NMDA) receptors enhance mechanical responses and voltage-dependent Ca^{2+} channels in rat DRG neurons through PK C Neuroscience 2004, 128, 347-357.

Chaban V. Visceral sensory neurons that innervate both uterus and colon express nociceptive TRPV1 and P2X3 receptors in rats. *Ethnicity and Disease* 2008 (18): Suppl. 2, 20-24.

Chaban V., Li J., McDonald J., Rapkin A., Micevych P. Estradiol attenuates ATP-induced increase of intracellular calcium through group II metabotropic glutamate B receptors in rat DRG neurons *Journal of Neuroscience Research* 2011, 89(11): 1707-10.

Cho T. and Chaban V. Interaction between P2X3 and estrogen receptors in ATP-mediated calcium signaling in mice sensory neurons. *Journal of Neuroendocrinology* 2012, (5):789-97.

Cho, T and Chaban V. Expression of P2X3 and TRPV1 receptors in DRG sensory neurons ERα/ERβ knock-out mice. *NeuroReport,* 20, 2012, 23(9):530-4.

Kannampalli P, Sengupta JN. Role of Principal Ionotropic and Metabotropic Receptors in Visceral Pain. *J Neurogastroenterol Motil.* 2015, 21(2): 147–158.

McCaffery M. Understanding your patient's pain. *Nursing*, 1980, 9: 26-31.

Melzack R. and Wall P. Pain mechanisms: a new theory. *Science,* 1965, 150: 971- 979.

Melzack, R. Evolution of the neuromatrix theory of pain. *Pain Pract.* 2005, 5: 85–94.

Melzak R. The future of pain. Nature Reviews Drug Discovery, 2008, 7: 629.

Chapter 2

Primary Afferent Nociceptors and Visceral Pain

Abstract

In this chapter author showed that modulation of visceral inputs of primary afferent nociceptors located in the afferent primary sensory neurons of dorsal root ganglia (DRG) accounts for the observed nociceptive changes in patients with chronic pelvic pain (CPP). For patients with Irritable Bowel Syndrome (IBS) the most common co-morbid diagnoses include CPP. CPP patients may initially have only one pain source in the pelvis, but a multitude of mechanisms involving the peripheral and central nervous system can lead to the development of painful sensations from other adjacent organs such as lower colonic pain associated with IBS and other viscera such as endometrium. Thus, in addition to central regulation it is important to understand new pathways how different modulators affect visceral nociception peripherally at the level of DRG.

Dorsal Root Ganglion As Potential Target in Modulation of Nociception

Direct activation of chemosensitive receptors and ion channels (discussed in previous chapter) on their peripheral terminals and modulation of neuronal excitability activates extrinsic primary afferent nerves. The cell bodies of primary visceral spinal afferent neurons are located in dorsal root ganglia (DRG). In humans, there are 31 right-and-left pairs of "mixed" spinal nerves carrying autonomic and sensorimotor information between the spinal cord and the periphery. These spinal nerves, formed from dorsal afferent sensory axons that became the dorsal rootlets and ventral efferent motor axons that became the ventral rootlets, emerge from the intervertebral neural foramina between adjacent vertebral segments and between the superior and inferior pedicles. As the dorsal sensory root fibers travel laterally, their processes connect with their cell bodies, which make up the DRG (Figure 2.1).

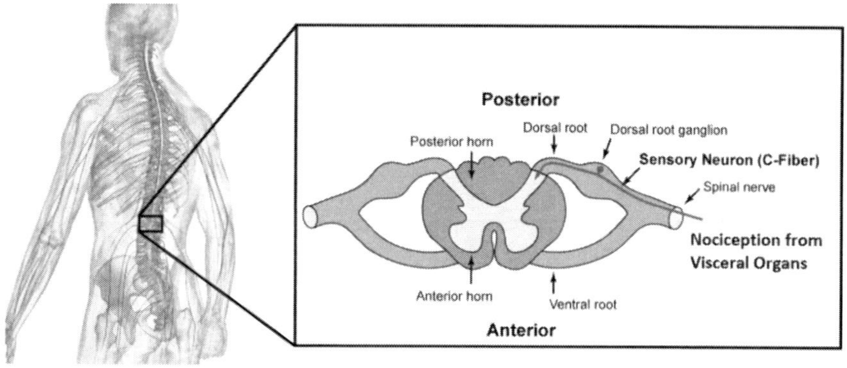

Figure 2.1. Structural characteristics of afferent nociceptive pathway from peripheral visceral organs via dorsal root ganglion to interneurons within dorsal horn of spinal cord.

Because DRG neurons have two branches that act as a single axon, a distal process and a proximal process, connected by a cell body as an offshoot, they are called pseudounipolar neurons. There are two major types of nociceptors, the small unmyelinated (C- fibers) and myelinated (Aδ- fibers) afferent neurons. The small polymodal C- fibers are responsible for the transmission of diffuse aching sensations. Their transmission is relatively slow (slow pain) and poorly localized. Transmission through the Aδ nociceptors is faster and well localized (sharp pain). Primary sensory afferent neurons form synapses with interneurons within dorsal horn of spinal cord forming contralateral spinothalamic tract, and then ascend to the cerebral cortex. Two divisions of spinothalamic tract carry nociceptive information to the cortex: the lateral neospinothalamic tract (for acute pain) and the medial paleospinothalamic tract (for dull and burning pain). The neospinothalamic tract carries information to the lateral thalamus and then projects to the primary somatosensory cortex to process specific nociceptive information. The paleospinothalamic tract carries information to the medial thalamus, brain stem, reticular formation, and hypothalamus and is responsible for pain reflexes with changes in endocrine and autonomic function, respiration, circulation. Nociceptive information is transmitted to primary somatosensory cortex for further processing. Descending efferent pathways and basal nuclei such as VM (ventromedial medulla) and PAG (periaqueductal gray) modulate or inhibit afferent pain signals within dorsal horn neurons. The cell DRG bodies, previously thought to be only metabolic storage "helpers" to peripheral processes, are now known to participate in the signaling process by sensing certain molecules and manufacturing other molecules that modulate these processes. There are several types of DRG neurons, classified by the size of the cell bodies and their function. Type A DRG neurons are large and are responsible for touch, vibration, and proprioception; type B neurons are small in size and are responsible for nociception. Histological studies estimate that the number of small neurons (type B) exceeds that of large neurons (type A) at a ratio of 71:29 (Kishi et al. 2002). Generally, nociceptors belong predominantly to small and medium size DRG neurons whose peripheral processes detect potentially damaging physical and chemical stimuli. The terminals of primary visceral afferent neurons are described as having no organs end or morphological specialization, but respond to different chemical stimuli. Visceral nociceptive C-fibers activated by ATP released by noxious stimuli from cells in target organs, have been implicated as mediators of noxious stimulus intensities (Burnstock 2000, 2001). ATP is a nucleoside triphosphate, is an end product of photophosphorelation and cellular respiration, and is the main unit of energy transfer within cells. ATP is also used by proteins and enzymes in a host of biosynthetic reactions, cell division, and motility. ATP is a ligand for the recently discovered new family of ion channels, the P2X family of ligand-gated ion channels, which are expressed by DRG nociceptive neurons (Chaban 2010). P2X3 mRNA is highly distributed within small C-fiber sensory nociceptors and their sensory neurons. Painful stimuli propagate to neurons within the DRG and then to the dorsal horn of the spinal cord. Alteration in signal transduction of primary afferent neurons can result in enhanced perception of the visceral sensation that is common in patients with different disorders resulting in elevated pain perception. Acute and recurrent chronic pelvic pain CPP and abdominal pain are illustrative examples of visceral pain that undergo primary afferent neurons sensitization (Giamberardino et al. 2010). Primary DRG neurons culture has been a useful model system for investigating sensory physiology and putative nociceptive signaling (Chaban et al. 2003). Small diameter DRGs (presumably nociceptors) in addition to purinergic P2X3 express vanilloid TRPV1, SP and metabotropic glutamate (mGluR) receptors (Chaban 2010; Chaban et al. 2011). Cultured lumbar-sacral (L4- S2) DRG neurons have been used for more than a decade in our laboratory to model the response of nociceptors to painful stimuli such as ATP (P2X3 receptor agonist) and capsaicin TRPV1 receptor agonist). Within the context of cross-sensitization hypothesis, inflammation sensitizes non-inflamed viscera that are innervated by the same DRG and/ or cross- sensitization occurs as a result of intra-DRG release of sensitizing mediators such as ATP or substance P in the DRG (Matsuka et al. 2001). Within the context of visceral nociception, nociceptor sensitization appear to be regulated by P2X3 and TRPV1. The primary sensory neuron starts in the neuron's peripheral receptive field, a region of the body in which a stimulus—as in injury or inflammation—alters the firing of the neuron, and ends within the CNS. Stimulation of the DRG may have both upstream and down- stream physiologic effects. Neuroactive agents (ATP, bradykinins, etc.) respond to changes in their environment, and influence neighboring cells, including DRG neurons (Cherkes et al. 2003). Therefore, DRG is a vibrant and active organ participating in the origination and modulation of physiological activity in response to environmental pressures. In response to injury or inflammation, a whole cascade of events occurs within and around DRG cell bodies, including changes in cytokine and chemokine production, up-regulation of immune factors, changes to surrounding glial cells, early and late genetic changes, and changes in Na^+, K^+, and Ca^{2+} ion channels (Krames 2015).

The role of the DRG in neuromodulation of visceral pain is a relatively new field of basic and clinical research. There is a considerable research to support the hypothesis that signal transduction mechanisms within the DRG contribute to modulation of nociception as well as development of chronic pain. Although it is generally accepted that each primary afferent neuron is a single sensory channel, several studies have challenged that view and demonstrate that a population of DRG neuron can innervate both the viscera and somatic tissues. When a repeated ATP (5 μM) stimulation was used within 5 min the $[Ca^{2+}]_i$ showed an increasing response (Figure 2.2B). Similarly, pre-treatment with substance P (10 μM) augmented the subsequent $[Ca^{2+}]_i$ response induced by ATP (Figure 2.2C). Thus, substance P or increasing amounts of ATP that signal nociception and sensitize response to ATP may be a good model to study cellular mechanism of peripheral sensitization (Chaban 2010). ATP plays a vital role in cellular metabolism as a potent extracellular signal. ATP transduces noxious stimuli by activating purinergic, ATP-gated P2X receptors on primary afferent fibers.

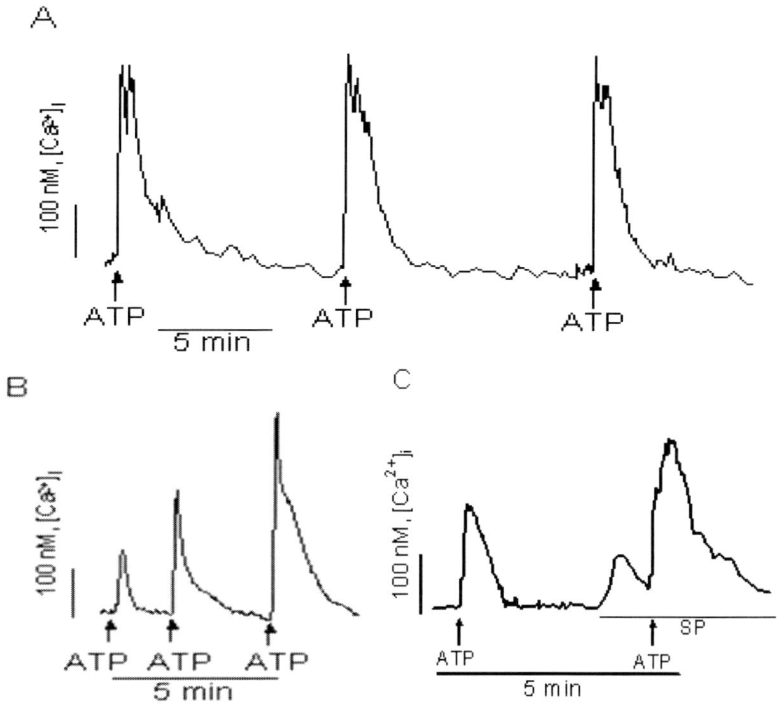

Figure 2.2. Sensitization of DRG neurons in vitro. A) Repeated ATP (10 μM) stimulation after 10 min wash-out with experimental medium produced reproducible $[Ca^{2+}]_i$ responses in DRG neurons (time and $[Ca^{2+}]_i$ indicated by bars). The trace is from a single neuron and shows features of typical responses with rapid rise after stimulation (indicated by arrow) followed by a slower recovery; B) Sensitization of $[Ca^{2+}]_i$ response to repeated stimulation with ATP (5 μM); C) Substance P (SP; 10 μM) increases ATP-induced $[Ca^{2+}]_i$ flux suggesting sensitization.

Opening of P2X channels results in membrane depolarization sufficient to trigger action potentials and Ca^{2+} influx through voltage-gated calcium channels (VGCC) associated with nociception. According to accepted theory pain, tissue irritation (mechanical distortion or inflammation) is due to ATP activation of high threshold nociceptors. The inflammatory process produces a number of mediators which activate nociceptors by interacting with ligand-gated ion channels or by sensitizing primary afferents. One mechanism for sensitization involves phosphorylation of ion channels and receptors including P2X and substance P. Sensitization accounts for a dramatically lowered nociceptive threshold to mechanical manipulation of the inflamed area. Within the context of the cross-sensitization hypothesis, inflammation can sensitizes non-inflamed viscera that are innervated by the same DRG. Cross-sensitization occurs as a result of intra-DRG release of sensitizing mediators such as ATP or substance P which we modeled in cultured DRG by repeated ATP or substance P and ATP stimulation. Visceral nociception and nociceptor sensitization appear to be regulated by ATP and substance P, thus, the DRG is an important site of visceral afferent convergence and cross-sensitization. Author of this book proposed two non-exclusive models for viscero-visceral cross-sensitization in the DRG (Chaban 2012, Figure 2.3).

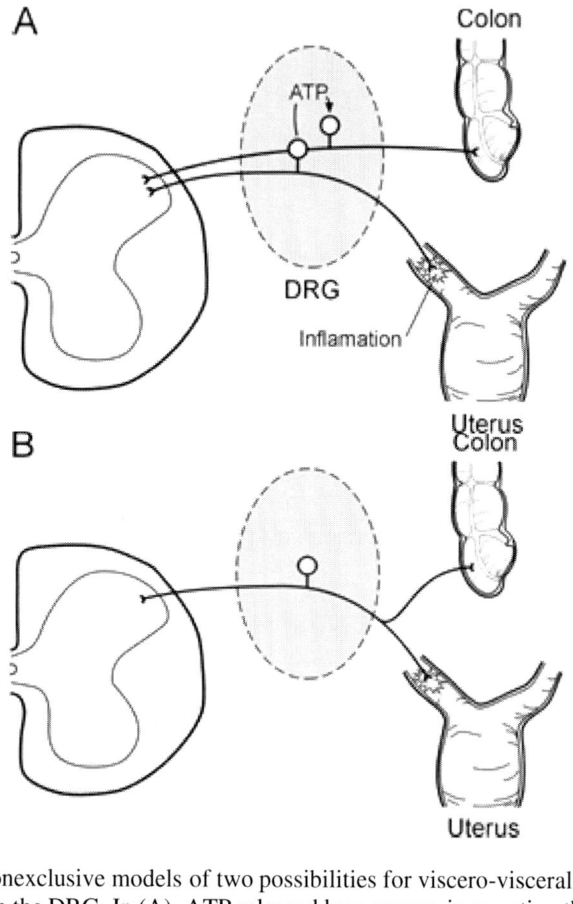

Figure 2.3. Nonexclusive models of two possibilities for viscero-visceral cross-sensitization in the DRG. In (A), ATP released by a neuron innervating the inflamed uterus acts on a neighboring neuron sensitizing its responses to colonic distention. In (B), the same neuron innervates the uterus and colon. Uterus inflammation directly sensitizes the neuron to colonic distention.

Chronic pain is persistent, lasting at least 3 to 6 months and related to tissue damage, inflammation, or anatomical or functional injury to nervous system predominantly via C neuron stimulation. Changes in nerve terminals, afferent fibers and then the CNS contribute to development of chronicity of pain. The physiological responses to chronic pain depend on the persistent or intermittent nature of pain. Intermittent pain produces response similar to acute pain, whereas persistent pain allows for physiological adaptation producing normal major vital signs such as heart and respiratory rates as well as normal blood pressure. However, even though the physiological responses are normal, the pain is not relieved. Living with pain requires constant attention to its earliest signs to avoid pain- provoking stimuli. The pain frequently does not respond to traditional therapy even when the cause is known. The nature of pain has been a subject of intense but still controversial research traditionally focusing on CNS. I hope to show the scientific community that the DRG is an active structure, which contradicts the long held belief that this ganglion was passive. The novel information from basic and clinical research should facilitate the translation of findings from the bench to bedside and from bedside to the bench. New hypotheses can be formed to conduct studies that should improve our understanding about the mechanisms of visceral pain and generate new forms of treatments for suffering patients.

References

Burnstock, G. P2X receptors in sensory neurons. *Br J Anaesth*, 2000, 84(4): 476-488.

Burnstock, G. Purine-mediated signaling in pain and visceral perception. *Trends Phannacol Sci,* 2001, 22(4):182-188.

Chaban V., Mayer E., Ennes H., Micevych P. Estradiol inhibits ATP-induced $[Ca^{2+}]_i$ increase in DRG neurons. *Neuroscience* 2003, 118 (6), 941-948.

Chaban V. Peripheral sensitization of sensory neurons. *Ethnicity and Disease* 2010 (20), Suppl. 1, 3-6.

Chaban V., Li J., McDonald J., Rapkin A., Micevych P. Estradiol attenuates ATP-induced increase of intracellular calcium through group II metabotropic glutamate B receptors in rat DRG neurons. *Journal of Neuroscience Research* 2011, 89(11): 1707-10.

Chaban V. Estrogen and visceral nociception at the level of primary sensory neurons. *Pain Research and Therapies* 2012, 1: pii: 960780.

Cherkes P, Hueng T, Pannicke T et al. The effects of axotomy on neurons and satellite glial cells in mouse trigeminal ganglion. *Pain* 2003; 110:290–298.

Giamberardino, M., Costantini A et al. Viscero-visceral hyperalgesia: characterization in different clinical models. *Pain,* 2010 151(2): 307-322.

Kishi M, Tanabe J, Schmelzer JD, Low PA. Morphometry of dorsal root ganglion in chronic experimental diabetic neuropathy. *Diabetes* 2002; 51: 819–824.

Krames E.S. The dorsal root ganglion in chronic pain and as a target for neuromodulation: a review. Neuromodulation 2015; 18: 24–32.

Matsuka, Y., J. K. Neubert, et al. Concurrent release of ATP and substance P within Guinea pig trigeminal ganglia in vivo. *Brain Res,* 2001 915(2): 248-255.

Chapter 3

Gender Differences in Visceral Nociception

Abstract

This chapter review the gender differences in nociceptive diseases observed in clinical practice. The prevalence of many functional disorders is much higher in female than male. The variations of symptoms and pain perception across the menstrual cycle and that sexual intercourse trigger symptoms in a large percentage of females diagnosed with functional syndromes such as Irritable Bowel Syndrome (IBS), Painful Bladder Syndrome (PBS), Chronic Pelvic Pain (CPP) and others suggest the involvement of sex steroids. Our studies showed that estrogen modulation of visceral inputs of primary afferent nociceptors located in the dorsal root ganglia (DRG) accounts for the observed changes in pain perception and symptoms observed during etiology of these functional pain syndromes. A multitude of mechanisms involving the peripheral and central nervous system can lead to the development of painful sensations from different adjacent organs. The localization of estrogen receptors in dorsal root ganglion (DRG) neurons strongly suggest that estradiol (E2) modulates visceral pain processing peripherally. E2 (both short-term and long-term exposure) significantly decreased the nociceptive signaling in viscerally-labeled DRG neurons. Thus, in addition to central regulation estrogen may affect nociception peripherally.

Nociceptive Pathways in Functional Disorders

A large body of literature supports the idea that estrogen modulates nociceptive responses in pelvic pain syndromes; however, whether this hormone is pro- or anti-nociceptive remains unresolved. Within the context of our hypothesis visceral nociception and nociceptor sensitization appear to be regulated by purinergic $P2X_3$ and vanilloid TRPV1 receptors (see Chapter 2) and 17β-estradiol modulates DRG neuron response to ATP (P2X agonist) and capsaicin (TRPV1 agonist) suggesting that visceral afferent nociceptors are modulated by estrogen in the DRG. 17-β estradiol (E2), the most common form of estrogen, acts on functional properties of $P2X_3$ and TRPV1 receptors in DRG neurons *in vitro*.

The localization of estrogen receptors (ER) in DRG neurons and the attenuation of ATP/capsaicin-induced intracellular calcium concentration $[Ca^{2+}]_i$ strongly suggest that E2 modulates visceral pain processing peripherally. Moreover, E2 appears to have different actions on nociceptive signaling depending on the input. Based on our data we propose that E2 can gate primary afferent response to increase or decrease nociception.

In women, pain symptoms and nociceptive thresholds vary with reproductive cycle and our previous data strongly suggest the role of estrogen receptors in modulating nociceptive signaling (Chaban 2011). 17β-estradiol (E2), the most potent estrogen of a group of endogenous estrogen steroids may be a causative factor inducing inflammation that contribute to the observed sex difference in visceral pain associated with functional pain syndromes. Most of the current literature pertains to specific functional syndromes defined by medical subspecialties. These include: irritable bowel syndrome: IBS (gastroenterology); chronic pelvic pain: CPP (gynecology); interstitial cystitis/painful bladder syndrome: IC/PBS (urology); fibromyalgia (rheumatology) and others. Many reports have described substantial overlaps between two or more of these syndromes (Malykhina 2007; Groover et al. 2009). Moreover, clinical presentations of functional syndromes lack a specific pathology in the affected organ but may respond to a viscero-visceral cross-sensitization in which increased nociceptive input from an inflamed organ (i.e., uterus) sensitizes neurons that receive convergent input from an unaffected organ (i.e., colon or bladder). The site of visceral cross-sensitivity is unknown.

Recent data from our laboratory and others showed that viscero-visceral cross-sensitization occurs in the dorsal root ganglion (DRG) where it is modulated by E2. Nociceptive transmitter ATP releases within sensory ganglia (Matsuka, 2008) suggest a site and mechanism for cross-sensitization, but depending on the prevailing conditions, E2 can have anti-nociceptive or pro-nociceptive actions.

The incidence of episodic or persistent visceral functional pain disorders such as IBS, IC/PBS, are 2-3 times more prevalent in women than men. Our hypothesis is that E2 modulation of cross-sensitization of visceral inputs in the DRG accounts for the observed changes in pain perception and symptoms in functional pain syndromes. E2 attenuation of ATP/capsaicin-induced $[Ca^{2+}]_i$ response, and decreased expression of P2X3 and TRPV1 receptors in estrogen receptor-α knockout (ERαKO) and estrogen receptor-β (ERβKO) knockout mice (Cho and Chaban 2012) strongly suggest that E2 modulates pain processing peripherally. Moreover, E2 appears to have different actions on nociceptive signaling depending on the input. Visceral nociceptive capsaicin-sensitive C-fibers are activated by ATP and excitatory amino acids that are released by noxious stimuli from cells in target organs (paracrine action), from afferent terminals themselves (autocrine action), or in sensory ganglia. In our studies we observed that DRG neurons innervating viscera have a greater $[Ca^{2+}]_i$ response to subsequent ATP and capsaicin and NMDA stimulation than somatic afferents (McRoberts et al. 2001) These observations indicate that viscerally-specific neurons express receptors with higher permeability to calcium, which can modulate transduction of nociceptive signals and suggest that visceral afferents are functionally different from somatic afferents . Sensitization of primary afferent neurons may play a role in the enhanced perception of visceral sensation leading to pain.

Mechanisms of peripheral sensitization may involve an increase in the excitability of the afferent nerves by molecules that decrease the excitation threshold. Sensitization can develop in response to inflammation. Phosphorylation-dependent modulation of the vanilloid receptor TRPV1 is one of the key mechanisms mediating the hyperalgesic effects of inflammatory mediators, such as prostaglandin E2 (PGE2) in sensory neurons (Schnizler et al. 2008). Significantly, inflammation dramatically alters TRPV 1 receptor-mediated transduction and purinoception by causing a several fold increase in ATP-activated currents, and enhances the expression of P2X receptors increasing neuronal hypersensitivity.

Inflammatory Activation of DRG Neurons

Number of molecules and neurotrophic factors are involved in hyperalgesia and overall sensory neuron sensitization. The inflammatory process produces mediators which activate nociceptors by interacting with ligand-gated ion channels or by sensitizing primary afferents. One mechanism for sensitization involves phosphorylation of ion channels and receptors including P2X3 and TRPV1 receptors. Inflammation does not change the percentage of total cells responding to ATP but sensitizes the ATP response by increasing the expression of P2X3. Thus, the greater behavioral sensitivity during the inflammation is due to a twofold to threefold increase in ATP responses suggesting that a small amount of ATP would evoke depolarization sufficient to elicit action potentials in DRG neurons. This pathological response arises from sensitization of DRG to external stimuli. Furthermore, inflamed tissues augment nociceptor responsiveness by acting on TRPV1. Gastrointestinal inflammation modulates the intrinsic properties of nociceptive dorsal root ganglia neurones, which innervate the GI tract and these changes are important in the genesis of abdominal pain and visceral hyperalgesia. Neurons exhibit hyperexcitability characterized by a decreased threshold for activation and increased firing rate. Inflammation upregulates the activity of N-methyl-D-aspartate receptors (NMDARs) in all DRG neurons within ganglia innervating viscera (Negri et al. 2006). Sensitization may also account for a lowered nociceptive threshold to mechanical manipulation of the inflamed area. Within the context of our cross-sensitization hypothesis, inflammation sensitizes non-inflamed viscera that are innervated by the same DRG and/or cross-sensitization occurs as a result of intra-DRG release of sensitizing mediators such as ATP within the DRG.

Estrogen Modulation of Nociception in PNS

Several lines of evidence indicate that E2 directly influence the functions of primary afferent neurons. Both subtypes of estrogen receptors (ERα and ERβ) are present in DRG neurons including the small-diameter putative nociceptors. In vitro, ATP-sensitive DRG neurons respond to E2, which correlated well with the idea that visceral afferents are E2 sensitive: i) visceral pain is affected by hormonal level in cycling females; ii) there are sex differences in the prevalence of functional disorders involving the viscera; and iii) putative visceral afferents fit into the population of DRG neurons that are sensitive to E2. These data suggest that in addition to CNS actions of E2, E2 can act in the periphery to modulate nociception.

ERα/ERβ receptors were traditionally envisioned as E2-activated transcription factors. However, more recent studies indicate that E2 has a multiplicity of actions: membrane, cytoplasmic and nuclear. E2 modulates cellular activity by altering ion channel opening, G-protein signaling, and activation of trophic factor-like signal transduction pathways. These effects have been ascribed to membrane-associated receptors. Moreover, estrogen receptors (ERs) are distributed in regions of the central and peripheral nervous system that mediate nociception. For example, ERs are expressed in dorsal horn neurons of the spinal cord and DRG neurons. Results from our laboratory and others indicate that E2 acts in DRG neurons to modulate L-type voltage-gated calcium channels (L-VGCC) and through group II metabotropic glutamate receptors. E2 has a significant role in modulating visceral sensitivity, indicating that E2 alterations in sensory processing may underlie sex-based differences in functional pain symptoms. However, reports of E2 modulation of visceral and somatic nociceptive sensitivity are inconsistent. Our previous studies showed that ATP (10 μM) induced $[Ca^{2+}]_i$ transients in 48% of small diameter DRG neurons in mice, a result similar to that observed in rat DRG neurons (53%) (Chaban and Micevych, 2005). A five minute incubation with E_2 (100 nM) inhibited ATP-induced $[Ca^{2+}]_i$ (137 $\pm$ 11.3 vs. 273 $\pm$ 12.4 nM, n = 8, $p < 0.05$, Figure 3.1). The effect of E_2 was similar in estrogen receptor-β knock out (ERβKO) mice DRG neurons (n = 7) (Figure 3.1C). However, in DRG neurons from estrogen receptor-α knock out (ERαKO) mice, E_2 did not block ATP-induced $[Ca^{2+}]_i$ suggesting that E_2 attenuation depends on ERα (n = 12) (Figure 3.1B). Estradiol- 17α had no effect on wild type (Wt), ERαKO or ERβKO mice.

Little is known about E2-mediated mechanisms in peripheral nervous system, but the fact that DRG neurons express ERs and respond to E2 treatment suggest that they are a potential target for mediating nociception. From a public health prospective, the outcome of this study will have a substantial impact on our knowledge of nociceptive functional diseases and help achieve a deeper understanding of gender differences presented in clinical aspects of these symptoms. Only a thorough understanding of the mechanism implicated in these phenomena can truly contribute to the designing of new and more efficient therapies.

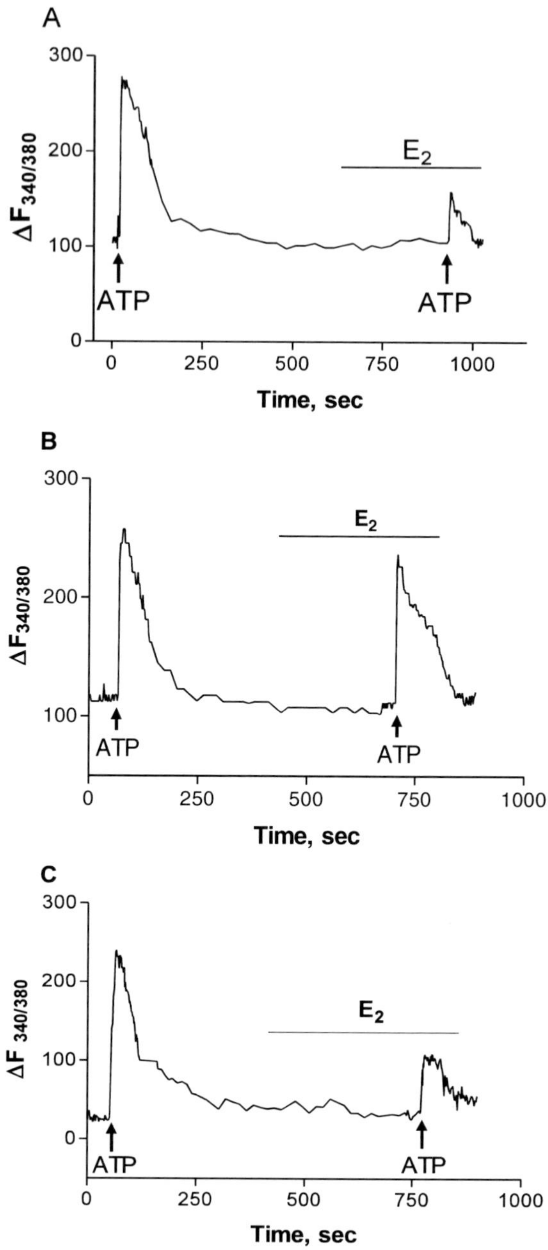

Figure 3.1. Effect of 17β- estradiol (E2, 100nM) on ATP-induced $[Ca^{2+}]_i$ flux in cultured DRG neurons from Wt (A), ERαKO (B) and ERβKO (C) mice. Duration of E2 in culture indicated by bars; addition of a pulse of ATP indicated by arrows.

Many illnesses affect women and men differently. Some disorders are more common in women, and some express themselves with different symptoms. Many studies confirmed that differences between the sexes exist in the prevalence and severity of a broad range of diseases, disorders and conditions. In the United States, pain accounts for nearly 20% of all primary health care visits. Proposed studies address a crucial question in women's health. Reaching further than the concrete basic science contribution, this project is a liaison between the basic science work and the clinical aspects that are addressed through other disciplines such as anesthesiology (pain management), gastroenterology and gynecology. A large body of literature supports the idea that E2 modulates nociceptive responses in pelvic pain syndromes; however, this mechanism remains unresolved. Within the context of our hypothesis E2 modulation of nociceptive response depends on the type of pain, its durations and the involvement of other nociceptive-mediated mechanisms. Visceral nociception appears to be regulated by ATP/capsaicin and E2 in the periphery at the level of DRG. The DRG is an important site of visceral afferent convergence and cross-sensitization.

References

Chaban, V. and P. Micevych, Estrogen receptor-alpha mediates estradiol attenuation of ATP-induced Ca^{2+} signaling in mouse dorsal root ganglion neurons. *J Neurosci Res*, 2005. 81(1): p. 31-7.

Chaban, V., Li, J., McDonald, J. S., Rapkin, A. and Micevych, P. 2011, *J. Neurosci. Res.,* 89, 1707-10.

Cho T. and Chaban V. Interaction between P2X3 and estrogen receptors in ATP-mediated calcium signaling in mice sensory neurons. *Journal of Neuroendocrinology* 2012, (5):789-97.

Grover, M., Herfarth, H. and Drossman, D. A. 2009, *Clin. Gastroenterol. Hepatol.,* 7, 48-53.

Malykhina, A. P. 2007, *Neuroscience,* 149, 660-72.

Matsuka, Y., Matsuka, Y., Ono, T., Iwase, H., Mitrirattanakul, S., Omoto, K. S., Cho, T., Lam, Y. Y., Snyder, B. and Spigelman, I. 2008, *Mol. Pain*, 4, 66.

McRoberts, J. A., Coutinho, S. V., Marvizón, J. C., Grady, E. F., Tognetto, M., Sengupta, J. N., Ennes, H. S., Chaban, V. V., Amadesi, S., Creminon, C.,

Lanthorn, T., Geppetti, P., Bunnett, N. W. and Mayer, E. A. 2001, *Gastroenterology,* 120, 1737-48.

Negri, L., Lattanzi, R., Giannini, E., Colucci, M., Margheriti, F., Melchiorri, P., Vellani, V., Tian, H., De Felice, M. and Porreca, F. 2006, *J. Neurosci.,* 26, 6716-27.

Schnizler, K., Shutov, L. P., Van Kanegan, M. J., Merrill, M. A., Nichols, B., McKnight, G. S., Strack, S., Hell, J. W. and Usachev, Y. M. 2008, *J. Neurosci.,* 28, 4904-17.

Chapter 4

Primary Nociceptors in Visceral Pain of Irritable Bowel Syndrome

Abstract

This chapter reviews the potential role of visceral nociceptors in etiology of Irritable Bowel Syndrome. The variations of symptoms and pain perception across the menstrual cycle and that sexual intercourse triggers symptoms in a large percentage of females with an Irritable Bowel Syndrome (IBS) patients suggest the involvement of sex steroids. Our studies suggest that estrogen modulation of visceral inputs of primary afferent nociceptors located in DRG accounts for the observed changes in pain perception and symptoms observed during etiology of this functional pain syndrome. The localization of estrogen receptors (ER) in DRG neurons and the attenuation of ATP-induce $[Ca^{2+}]_i$ strongly suggest that 17β-estradiol (E2) modulates visceral pain peripherally. Multitude of mechanisms involving the peripheral and central nervous system can lead to the development of painful sensations from other adjacent organs such as lower colonic pain associated with IBS.

Transduction of Nociceptive Signals

Primary afferents transmit information about chemical or mechanical stimulation from the periphery to the spinal cord. Nociceptors are small to medium size DRG neurons whose peripheral processes detect potentially damaging physical and chemical stimuli. ATP has emerged as a putative signal for visceral pain. ATP is released by distention of the viscera and tissue damage (for review see (Burnstock 2001). Visceral nociceptive C-fibers are activated by ATP and excitatory amino acids that are released by noxious stimuli from cells in target organs (paracrine action), from afferent terminals themselves (autocrine action), or in sensory ganglia (Matsuka, Neubert et al. 2001). In our studies we observed that DRG neurons innervating viscera have a greater $[Ca^{2+}]_i$ response to subsequent NMDA stimulation than somatic afferents (McRoberts, Coutinho et al. 2001). This observation indicates that these neurons express receptors with higher permeability to Ca^{2+}, which can modulate transduction of nociceptive signals and suggests that visceral afferents are functionally different from somatic afferents. Sensitization of primary afferent neurons to stimulation may play a role in the enhanced perception of visceral sensation and pain. Pain in women with endometriosis or abdominal pain from IBS is all visceral pain sensations that may result in part from sensitization (Berkley, Cason et al. 2001; Mayer, Naliboff et al. 2001). Mechanisms of peripheral sensitization may involve increased transduction that is secondary to repeated stimulation or an increase in the excitability of the afferent nerves by molecules that decrease the excitation threshold (Zimmermann 2001). Sensitization can develop in response to inflammation. Although basic mechanisms are probably similar, visceral nociception differs from the pathophysiology of cutaneous hyperalgesia (Chang and Heitkemper 2002).

ATP plays vital roles in cellular metabolism and as an extracellular signal. ATP transduces noxious stimuli by activating purinergic, ATP-gated P2X receptors on primary afferent fibers. Opening of P2X channels results in membrane depolarization sufficient to trigger action potentials and Ca2+ influx through define VGCC associated with nociception. According to this theory pain of tissue irritation (mechanical distortion or inflammation) is due to ATP activation of high threshold nociceptors (Burnstock 2001). The predominant ATP receptor in small diameter nociceptive DRG neurons is the P2X3. P2X3-null mice have reduced pain-related behavior in response to noxious stimuli (Cockayne, Hamilton et al. 2000). Significantly, inflammation dramatically alters purinoception by causing a several fold increase in ATP-activated currents, alters the voltage dependence of P2X receptors, and enhances the expression of P2X receptors increasing neuronal hypersensitivity (Xu and Huang 2002).

The inflammatory process produces a number of mediators which activate nociceptors by interacting with ligand-gated ion channels or by sensitizing primary afferents. One mechanism for sensitization involves phosphorylation of ion channels and receptors including P2X receptors (Dai, Fukuoka et al. 2004). P2X receptor function is enhanced by a number of agents including ATP and substance P. Inflammation does not change the percentage of total cells responding to ATP but sensitizes the ATP response and increases the expression of P2X2 and P2X3 (Xu and Huang 2002). Thus, the increased behavioral sensitivity during the inflammation is due to a twofold to threefold increase in ATP responses suggesting that a small amount of ATP would evoke depolarization sufficient to elicit action potentials in DRG neurons (Xu and Huang 2002). This pathological response arises from sensitization of DRG and dorsal horn neurons to external stimuli. Sensitization accounts for a dramatically lowered nociceptive threshold to mechanical manipulation of the inflamed area. Within the context of the cross-sensitization hypothesis, inflammation can sensitizes non-inflamed viscera that are innervated by the same DRG. Cross-sensitization occurs as a result of intra-DRG release of sensitizing mediators such as ATP or substance P in the DRG (Matsuka, Neubert et al. 2001) and is modeled in cultured DRG by repeated ATP or substance P and ATP stimulation.

Estrogen Modulation of Nociception in Primary Afferent Neurons

Sex hormones and E2, in particular, may directly influence the functions of primary afferent neurons. Both subtypes of estrogen receptors (ERα and ERβ) are present in small-diameter DRG neurons (Papka and Storey-Workley 2002). While several actions of E2 have been demonstrated in the nervous system, the mechanisms of E2 pain modulation remain unclear. ERs were traditionally envisioned as E2-activated transcription factors. However, E2 has a multiplicity of actions: membrane, cytoplasmic and nuclear (reviewed in (Chaban, Li et al. 2011). E2 modulates cellular activity by altering ion channel opening, G-protein signaling, and activation of tropic factor-like signal transduction pathways (Chaban, Mayer et al. 2003). These effects have been ascribed to membrane-associated receptors. Relevant to the present proposal, ERs are distributed in regions of the central and peripheral nervous system that mediate nociception. For example, ERs are expressed in dorsal horn neurons of the spinal cord (Chaban 2010) and DRG neurons (Papka, Storey-Workley et al. 2001). Results from our laboratory (Chaban, Mayer et al. 2003) and others (Lee, Chai et al. 2002) indicate that E2 acts in neurons to modulate L-type VGCC.

In DRGs, ERα mRNA expression is primarily in small diameter, presumptively nociceptive neurons (Papka and Storey-Workley 2002). Distribution of ERs in small diameter DRG neurons is similar in both males and females. Several indirect pieces of evidence suggest that visceral afferents are E2 sensitive: i) visceral pain is affected by hormonal level in cycling females (Traub and Murphy 2002); ii) there are sex differences in the prevalence of functional disorders involving the viscera; and iii) putative visceral afferents (McRoberts, Coutinho et al. 2001) fit into the population of DRG neurons that are sensitive to E2 (Chaban, Mayer et al. 2003; Chaban, Li et al. 2011).

Most of the published reports in the area of sex and hormone-related differences in pain have addressed the modulatory effect of E2 on CNS mechanisms of nociception. Many studies demonstrate that E2 has a significant role in modulating visceral sensitivity, indicating that E2-alterations in sensory processing may underlie sex-based differences in functional pain symptoms (Al-Chaer and Traub 2002). However, reports of E2 modulation of visceral and somatic nociceptive sensitivity are inconsistent. For example, elevated E2 levels have been reported to increase the threshold to cutaneous stimuli but decrease the percentage of escape responses to ureteral calculosis (Bradshaw and Berkley 2002). Nociceptive sensitivity appears to increase when E2 levels are elevated. Indeed in most clinical studies, women report more severe pain levels, more frequent pain and longer duration of pain than men (Fillingim and Edwards 2001).

One prominent way E2 modulates neuronal excitability is through interactions with opioid systems (Sinchak and Micevych 2003). E2 modulates both the classic, anti-nociceptive opioids (e.g., enkephalins, β-endorphin and the pro-nociceptive nociceptin/orphanin systems. Nociceptin is the endogenous ligand for the opioid receptor-like orphanin receptor-1 (ORL1). In the hypothalamus and limbic system E2 increases nociceptin mRNA expression (Sinchak and Micevych 2003). Moreover, E2 reduces the efficacy of MOP agonist inhibition of nociceptive response to cervical distension in rats and the response to uterine cervical distension (Sandner-Kiesling and Eisenach 2002). Additionally, E2 attenuates the ability of MOP agonists to hyperpolarize hypothalamic neurons. These results are congruent with reports that sex steroids appear to mediate differential responses to opiate analgesics in men and women (Zubieta, Smith et al. 2002).

Many E2 actions appear to be mediated through a membrane ER. Membrane ERs are coded by the same transcripts as those that code intracellular ERα and ERβ in transfected cell and in DRG neurons. Membrane ERs have several features that distinguish them from intracellular receptors: time of activation, dose, and that membrane impermeable constructs mimic the effect of E2. Overall, based on our previous studies, we hypothesize that E2 can be anti-nociceptive, but under certain conditions, such as those associated with opioid anti-nociception, E2 becomes pro-nociceptive by blocking anti-nociceptive opioid input.

One of the explanations for the etiology of functional disorders such as Irritable Bowel Syndrome (IBS) can be that a subset of sensory neurons can receive an input from different visceral organs. To test this hypothesis retrograde labeling was used to identify cultured DRG neurons innervating the uterus or colon (as described in (Papka, Storey-Workley et al. 2001)). Briefly, the colon was exposed by abdominal incision and 2 μl of a 4% solution of Fluorogold (Fluorochrome, Englewood, CO) was injected into the muscle wall of descending colon. Animals were allowed to survive for 2 weeks and DRG were harvested. Approximately 10% of DRG (T12-S2) neurons innervated viscera (McRoberts, Coutinho et al. 2001). Labeled DRGs had responses that suggested functional NMDA, VR1, mechano- and opioid receptors. To label uterine afferents, tertramethylrhodamine (TMR, Molecular Probes, Eugene, OR) was injected the myometrium of the uterus. Up to 50% neurons were labeled with TMR in L1-S1 levels. Both dyes were injected into respective locations of the same animal (Figure 4.1). The same primary afferent may innervate both the uterus and the colon, and it is plausible that this population of dichotomizing neurons plays a vital role in the mechanism of nociceptive transduction at the level of primary afferent neurons. DRG neurons in vitro is a well-accepted model for examine primary afferent response to nociceptive and anti-nociceptive signals (McRoberts et al. 2001; Chaban, Mayer et al. 2003). Our studies tested the hypothesis that within lumbosacral segments, DRG neurons innervating visceral structures will respond to E2 more frequently than cutaneous afferents. Under fluorescent illumination we were able to distinguish visceral (uterine and colonic) DRG neurons based on their retrogradely transported dyes. Such an observation suggests that DRG neurons innervating the uterus and colon may have a greater percentage of ER expressing neurons or ERs in visceral afferents are more tightly coupled to signal transduction machinery.

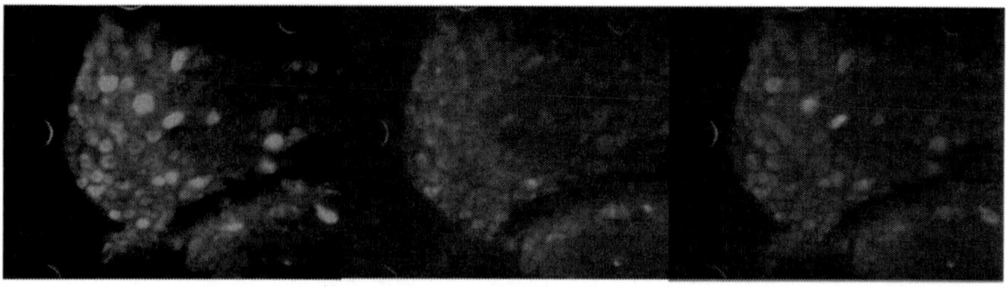

Figure 4.1. Retrogradely labeled DRG neurons following injections of Fluorogold (yellow) into the distal colon (left picture) and TMR (red) in the uterine cervix (middle picture) ; DRG labeled with Flourogold (colon) and TMR (uterine) dyes co-localized (orange) in the DRG neurons at the levels where neurons projected from the colon (L1, L2 and L6) as indicated in (right picture).

The DRG is an important site of visceral afferent convergence and cross-sensitization. We have demonstrated that E2, the most common form of estrogen act on functional properties of P2X receptors in DRG neurons in vitro. The localization of ER in DRG neurons and the attenuation of ATP-induce $[Ca^{2+}]_i$ strongly suggest that E2 modulates visceral pain processing peripherally. Moreover, E2 appears to have different actions on nociceptive signaling depending on the input. Adult DRG neurons in short-term culture retain the expression of P2X receptors which mediate the response to putative nociceptive signals. They continue to respond to ER agonists mimicking in vivo activation. An important advantage is that these neurons can be studied apart from endogenous signals. Our data clearly showed the new role of nociceptors in pathophysiological aspects of chronic pelvic pain and potential way of designing future therapies.

References

Al-Chaer, E. D. and R. J. Traub Biological basis of visceral pain: recent developments. *Pain* 2002, 96(3): 221-225.

Berkley, K. J., A. Cason, et al. Vaginal hyperalgesia in a rat model of endometriosis. *Neurosci Lett*, 2001, 306(3): 185-188.

Bradshaw, H. B. and K. J. Berkley Estrogen replacement reverses ovariectomy-induced vaginal hyperalgesia in the rat. *Maturitas,* 2002, 41(2): 157-165.

Burnstock, G. Purine-mediated signalling in pain and visceral perception." *Trends Pharmacol Sci*, 2001, 22(4): 182-188.

Chaban, V., J. Li, et al. Estradiol attenuates the adenosine triphosphate-induced increase of intracellular calcium through group II metabotropic glutamate receptors in rat dorsal root ganglion neurons. *J Neurosci Res*, 2011, 89(11): 1707-1710.

Chaban, V. V., E. A. Mayer, et al. Estradiol inhibits ATP-induced intracellular calcium concentration increase in dorsal root ganglia neurons. *Neuroscience,* 2003, 118(4): 941-948.

Chang, L. and M. M. Heitkemper Gender differences in irritable bowel syndrome. *Gastroenterology,* 2002 123(5): 1686-1701.

Cockayne, D. A., S. G. Hamilton, et al. Urinary bladder hyporeflexia and reduced pain-related behaviour in P2X3-deficient mice. *Nature,* 2000, 407(6807): 1011-1015.

Dai, Y., T. Fukuoka, et al. Contribution of sensitized P2X receptors in inflamed tissue to the mechanical hypersensitivity revealed by phosphorylated ERK in DRG neurons. *Pain*, 2004, 108(3): 258-266.

Fillingim, R. B. and R. R. Edwards The association of hormone replacement therapy with experimental pain responses in postmenopausal women. *Pain*, 2001, 92(1-2): 229-234.

Lee, D. Y., Y. G. Chai, et al. 17Beta-estradiol inhibits high-voltage-activated calcium channel currents in rat sensory neurons via a non-genomic mechanism. *Life Sci,* 2002, 70(17): 2047-2059.

Matsuka, Y., J. K. Neubert, et al. Concurrent release of ATP and substance P within guinea pig trigeminal ganglia in vivo. *Brain Res*, 2001 915(2): 248-255.

Mayer, E. A., B. D. Naliboff, et al. Basic pathophysiologic mechanisms in irritable bowel syndrome. *Dig Dis*, 2001, 19(3): 212-218.

McRoberts, J. A., S. V. Coutinho, et al. Role of peripheral N-methyl-D-aspartate (NMDA) receptors in visceral nociception in rats. *Gastroenterology*, 2001, 120(7): 1737-1748.

Papka, R. E. and M. Storey-Workley Estrogen receptor-alpha and -beta coexist in a subpopulation of sensory neurons of female rat dorsal root ganglia." *Neurosci Lett,* 2002, 319(2): 71-74.

Sandner-Kiesling, A. and J. C. Eisenach Estrogen reduces efficacy of mu- but Not kappa-opioid agonist inhibition in response to uterine cervical distension. *Anesthesiology,* 2002, 96(2): 375-379.

Sinchak, K. and P. Micevych Visualizing activaiton of opioid circuits by internalization of G protein-coupled receptors. *Molecular Neurobiology,* 2003, 27(2): 197-222.

Traub, R. J. and A. Murphy Colonic inflammation induces fos expression in the thoracolumbar spinal cord increasing activity in the spinoparabrachial pathway. *Pain*, 2002, 95(1-2): 93-102.

Xu, G. Y. and L. Y. Huang Peripheral inflammation sensitizes P2X receptor-mediated responses in rat dorsal root ganglion neurons. *J Neurosci*, 2002, 22(1): 93-102.

Zimmermann, M. Pathobiology of neuropathic pain. *Eur J Pharmacol*, 2001, 429(1-3): 23-37.

Zubieta, J. K., Y. R. Smith, et al. Mu-opioid receptor-mediated antinociceptive responses differ in men and women. *J Neurosci*, 2002, 22(12): 5100-5107.

Chapter 5

Nociception of Endometriosis

Abstract

This chapter review the basic process of endometriosis and potential role of visceral nociceptors in etiology of this disease. The mechanism of endometriosis-induced nociceptive signaling is poorly understood and in some cases pain can be exacerbated by co-morbidity with other chronic pelvic pain syndromes such as irritable bowel syndrome, painful bladder syndrome, vulvodynia and fibromyalgia. Visceral pain is the main concern for patients diagnosed with endometriosis. Within the context of cross-sensitization hypothesis, inflammation sensitizes non-inflamed viscera that are innervated by the same DRG and/or cross-sensitization occurs as a result of intra-DRG release of sensitizing mediators such as ATP or substance P in the DRG. This mechanism can provide a possible explanation of noception associated with endometriosis.

Etiology of Endometriosis

Endometrial tissues outside the uterus can cause severe pain and this pain can be diminished with therapies that suppress estrogen production (Berkley, Rapkin et al. 2005). It has also been shown that ectopic implants develop sensory nerve supply both in women and in animal models of endometriosis. Sensory input arriving from the visceral organ to the spinal cord divergences at the level of primary sensory neurons which further transmit considerable information from periphery to the central nervous system. Visceral pain may be manifestation from a single organ such as uterus or may arise from algogenic conditions affecting more than one organ (Malykhina 2007). This type of pain is important not only because it is difficult to diagnose its clinical conditions but also for its therapeutic implications. It is quite possible to modulate pain from one viscus to another. Recent study by Giamberardino and others showed that the treatment of the endometriotic lesions results in the improvement of spontaneous and referred urinary symptoms (Giamberardino, Costantini et al. 2010).

Cross-sensitization in the pelvis implies the transmission of noxious stimuli from one organ to another through an adjacent normal structure resulting in functional (rarely organic) changes. Pelvic organ cross-sensitization is considered as one of the factors contributing to chronic pelvic pain (Pezzone, Liang et al. 2005). Assessing the impact of the pain on various domains of a patient's existence has become an important focus in the clinical management. Most women with complaints of pelvic pain will undergo laparoscopy to both diagnose and treat these diseases, but laparoscopy is often is unsuccessful due to lack of intraperitoneal pathology or altered pain processing. Pain out of proportion to identifiable pathology is the most immediate and dramatic consequence of disorders associated with chronic pelvic pain (CPP) and is responsible for a highly negative impact on quality of life and substantial workforce loss.

There is often no clear relationship between the severity of the chronic pelvic pain and pathology in the pelvic viscera, including reproductive tract (ovaries and uterus). It is still poorly understood how endometriosis is associated with pain symptoms in different organs and how this nociceptive signaling is ameliorated by a hypoestrogenic state. One of the possible explanation can be that endometrial implants' sensory nerve supply and its potentially estradiol-modulated influence on the nociception. Several researchers have investigated the presence of nerve fibers in endometriotic lesions in both human and animal study. Using different types of specific immunohistochemical neuronal markers such as substance P (SP) and CGRP (sensory nerve fiber markers) in human peritoneal endometriotic lesions from women with visually and biopsy proven endometriosis, investigators has demonstrated multiple, small unmyelinated nerve fibers are present in peritoneal endometriotic lesions, and these peritoneal endometriotic lesions contain both Aδ and C nerve fibers. Accumulating evidence has shown these nerve fibers may play a critical role in pain production in patients with endometriosis, and a close histological relationship has been identified between these nerve fibers and endometriosis associated pain. Tulandi et al.

(2001) reported that the distance between endometriotic glands and nerve fibers in endometriotic lesions from women with pain was closer than in women with no pain. The density of nerve fibers in peritoneal endometriotic lesions was much greater than in normal peritoneum in women with no endometriosis. The nerve fiber density in endometriotic lesions can be markedly reduced by hormonal drugs such as GnRH analogues and combined oral contraceptives, which have been used efficaciously to treat endometriosis-associated pain, indicating that modulation of these nerve fibers might alter pelvic nociception. The fact that peritoneal endometriotic lesions are innervated by sensory Aδ, sensory C nerve fibers raises the intriguing questions, what kind of role do these nerve fibers play in the mechanisms by which endometriotic lesions produce pain and hyperalgesia, and how do they modulate pain perception in these condition? The demonstration of Aδ and C sensory fiber innervations to peritoneal endometriotic lesions, suggesting these innervations contributes to both visceral hyperalgesia and pelvic pain that occur in patients with endometriosis brings up the interesting questions, how do these sensory fibers transmit and modulate visceral nociception in endometriosis? Immunohistochemical staining of these nerve fibers in endometriosis showed co-localization of SP, CGRP, implicating SP and CGRP might be involved in modulation of visceral nociception. Endometriosis is an inflammatory disease, which are known to contain pro-inflammatory cytokines, prostaglandins, and other neuroactive agents that could readily activate the CGRP- and SP-positive C-fiber nociceptive afferents found in the endometriotic lesions. When these sensory nerve fibers are stimulated by inflammatory substances, neurotransmitters such as SP, CGRP can be secreted from sensory nerve endings. SP and CGRP can contribute to the inflammatory response by causing vasodilation, plasma extravasation and cellular infiltration by interacting with endothelial cells, arterioles, mast cells, neutrophils and immune cells. SP can also act on mast cells in the vicinity of sensory nerve endings to evoke de-granulation and the release of TNF-α, histamine, PGD2 and leukotriene, providing a positive feedback. CGRP has a wide range of biological activities, including sensory transmission, regulation of glandular secretion, and inhibiting SP degradation by a specific endopeptidase to enhance SP release, thereby amplifying the effects.

DRG neurons can be activated or modulated by the activation of chemosensitive receptors on peripheral terminals and ATP has been implicated in sensory transduction of noxious stimuli by activating purinergic P2X receptors. Once released into the intercellular areas, the action of ATP is mediated by primarily P2X3 receptors which are expressed on primary afferent fibers and cell bodies within DRG (Burnstock 2001). The capsaicin-sensitive primary afferent neurons of small- and medium-diameter neurons mediate nociceptive-like behaviors suggesting that TRPV1 expressing neurons are nociceptors. Activation of P2X3 and TRPV1 receptors results in the depolarization and opening of voltage-gated Ca2+channels (VGCC) (Koshimizu, Van Goor et al. 2000). A sensation of pain is produced by depolarization of the peripheral nerve terminals.

The terminals of primary visceral afferent neurons are described as having no organs end or morphological specialization, but respond to different chemical stimuli. Visceral nociceptive C-fibers activated by ATP released by noxious stimuli from cells in target organs, have been implicated as mediators of noxious stimulus intensities (Burnstock 2001). Alteration in signal transduction of primary afferent neurons can result in enhanced perception of the visceral sensation that is common in patients with different disorders resulting in elevated pain perception. Peripheral sensitization can develop in response to sustain stimulation, inflammation, and nerve injury. Endometriosis is currently defined as a chronic functional syndrome characterized by recurring symptoms of abdominal discomfort or pain. In the contest to visceral pain, the TRPV1 receptor is a sensory neuron-specific cation channel which belongs to the transient receptor potential subfamily 1 and plays an important role in transporting thermal and inflammatory pain signals. Evidence for TRPV1's role is that mice lacking TRP1R gene have deficits in thermal- or inflammatory-induced hyperalgesia.

E2 can modulate cellular activity by altering ion channel opening and second messenger signaling by stimulating G-proteins, the signal transduction pathways traditionally associated with membrane receptor activation. Many of these effects have been ascribed to membrane-associated receptors. Most of the published reports about sex and hormone-related differences in pain have addressed the modulatory effect of E2 on CNS mechanisms of nociception, however, reports of E2 modulation of visceral and somatic nociceptive sensitivity are inconsistent. Indeed in most clinical studies, women report more severe pain levels, more frequent pain and longer duration of pain than men. E2 acting on primary afferent nociceptors modulates the response to pro- and anti-nociceptive signals. Within the context of our cross-sensitization hypothesis, inflammation sensitizes non-inflamed viscera that are innervated by the same DRG and/or cross-sensitization occurs as a result of intra-DRG release of sensitizing mediators such as ATP or substance P in the DRG (Chaban 2008; Chaban 2010).

Role of P2X3 and TRPV1 Receptors in Estrogen-Induced Nociceptive Signaling in Sensory Neurons

In our study we have used 6~8 week female C57BL/6J, B6.129P2-Esr1tm1Ksk/J, and B6.129P2-Esr2tm1Unc/J mice were obtained the Jackson Laboratory (Bar Harbor, ME, USA). Upon arrival, mice were group housed in microisolator caging and maintained on a 12-h light/dark cycle in a temperature-controlled environment with access to food and water ad libitum. To test whether estrogen receptor α (ERα) or estrogen receptor β (ERβ) are involved in estradiol (E2)-induced modification of $[Ca^{2+}]_i$ Wile type (Wt), estrogen receptor alpha knock-out (ERαKO) and estrogen receptor beta knock-out (ERβKO) mice were used. The wild type, ERαKO and ERβKO mice were allowed to recover for two weeks. The isolation procedure and primary culture of mouse lumbosacral DRG has been published in detail (Chaban, Mayer et al. 2003). DRG tissues were obtained from c57/black 6J (The Jackson Laboratory; 30 g), ERαKO and ERβKO (Taconic; 20 g) transgenic types. Briefly, lumbosacral adult DRGs (level L1-S1) from Wt, ERαKO and ERβKO mice were collected under sterile technique and placed in ice-cold medium Dulbecco's Modified Eagle's Medium (DMEM; Sigma Chemical Co., St. Louis, MO). Adhering fat and connective tissue was removed and each DRG were minced with scissors and placed immediately in a medium consisting of 5 ml of DMEM containing 0.5 mg/ml of trypsin (Sigma, type III), 1 mg/ml of collagenase (Sigma, type IA) and 0.1 mg/ml of DNAase (Sigma, type III) and kept at 37°C for 30 minutes with agitation. After dissociation of the cell ganglia, soybean trypsin inhibitor (Sigma, type III) was used to terminate cell dissociation. Cell suspensions were centrifuged for one minute at 1000 rpm and the cell pellets were resuspended in DMEM supplemented with 5% fetal bovine serum, 2 mM glutamine-penicillin-streptomycin mixture, 1 μg/ml DNAase and 5 ng/ml NGF (Sigma). Cells were placed on Matrigel® (Invitrogen)-coated 15-mm coverslips (Collaborative Research Co., Bedford, PA) and kept at 37° C in 5% CO2 incubator for 24 hrs, given fresh media and maintained in primary culture until used for experimental procedures.

The expressions of TRPV1 and of P2X3 receptors in L1~S1 DRGs were studied by using Western blot analyses. Tissues from wild type (C57BL/6J), ERαKO, and ERβKO mice were quick frozen in tubes on dry ice during collection. L1~S1 DRG were combined, homogenized by mechanical disruption in ice-cold RIPA buffer plus protease inhibitors and incubated on ice for 30 minutes. Homogenates were then spun at 5000 g for 15 minutes and supernatants collected. Total protein was determined on the supernatants using the BCA microtiter method (Pierce, Rockford, Ill., USA). Samples containing equal amounts of protein (40μg) were electrophoresed under denaturing conditions using Novex Mini-cell system (San Diego, Calif., USA) and reagents (NuPage 4–12% Bis-Tris gel and MOPS running buffer). After electrophoretic transfer onto nitrocellulose membrane using the same system, the membrane was blocked with 5% non-fat dry milk (NFDM) in 25 mM TRIS buffered saline, pH 7.2, plus Tween 20 (TBST) for 1 hour at room temperature, followed by incubation with polyclonal rabbit antibody against TRPV1-N terminus (1:1000, Neuromics) and P2X3 receptor (1:1000, Neuromics) for overnight at 4oC. The membrane was then washed in culture midium, and incubated with secondary antibody, HRP conjugated and rabbit IgG (Santa Cruz Biotechnology) at 1:5,000 in the same buffer for 2 hours at room temperature. Following a final wash in TBST without NFDM, the membrane was incubated with ECL+ (Amersham, Arlington Heights, Ill., USA) substrate for HRP. Membranes were probed with primary antibody and corresponding secondary antibodies, signals were scanned and quantified by Image J version 1.28U and NIH Image 1.60 scan software. Following enhanced chemiluminescence (ECL) detection of proteins, the membranes were stripped and rehybridized with β-actin antibody as a loading control. At least three independent cell preparations were used.

DRG tissues were obtained from C57/black 6J (The Jackson Laboratory; 30 g), ERαKO and ERβKO (Taconic; 20 g) transgenic types. Following decapitation, DRG from bilateral spinal levels L1-S2 were removed and fixed in 4% paraformaldehyde for overnight at 4°C. DRGs were rinsed in Delbecco's Phosphate Buffered Saline (DPBS) before cryoprotection in sucrose (20%, 4°C) for two days, after which excess liquid was removed. DRG were quick snap frozen in 2-methylbutane, and store them at -70°C. Each DRG was mounted in Tissue-Tek® OCT embedding medium (Sakura Finetek), and sectioned at -20°C in a MICROM H505E cryostat. Sections were cut at 20μm and store 4°C until required. Sections of DRGs were collected in PBS. Endogenous tissue peroxidase activity was quenched by soaking the sections for 10 min in 3% hydrogen peroxide solution in 0.01 M PBS. The specimens were washed and then treated for 60 min in blocking solution, 0.01 M PBS containing 0.5% Triton X-100 and 1% normal donkey serum (NDS) at room temperature. They were processed for wild type (n=4), ERαKO (n=4), or ERβKO (n=4) immunohistochemistry by the free floating method using polyclonal rabbit TRPV1 antibody (1:50000, Neuromics) or P2X3 receptor antibody (1:15000, Neuromics) for overnight at 4°C, washed in 0.01 M phosphate-buffered saline (PBS) and 0.01M Tris Buffered Saline (TBS), followed by incubation in solutions of donkey anti-rabbit fluorophore-conjugated secondary antibodies (1:200, Invitrogen) in 0.01M Tris Buffered Saline (TBS) for 3 hours at room temperature. Cells showing no apparent or only faint membrane/intracellular labeling were considered to be negative for TRPV1 or P2X3. TRPV1-positive cells included those with strong plasma membrane labeling that formed a discernible clustered pattern, and those with strong intracellular labeling that formed a punctuate pattern. Some neurons showed both strong plasma membrane and intracellular labeling. P2X3-positive neurons showed diffuse membrane/ intracellular labeling. Mounted sections were air dried and coverslipped with Aqua Poly Mount (Polisciences, Warrington, PA). Images from at least three sections in each level were taken using Leica DMLB M130X microscope. The total numbers of DRG neurons expressing TRPV1 and P2X3 were counted. TRPV1- or P2X3-positive neurons were categorized according to their labeling patterns and were expressed as a percentage of the total number of TRPV1- or P2X3-positive cells. Immunohistochemical signal percent was measured by computerized image analysis (Image Pro-Plus, Media Cybernetics, Silver Spring, MD, USA). P2X3 and TRPV1 receptors expression were examined by western blot analysis of lysates from wild type, ERαKO, and ERβKO DRG tissues using a P2X3 specific primary antiserum. An intense band representing a ~64 kDa protein (P2X3) and a ~130 kDa (TRPV1) was seen in DRG lysates from wild type animals. There was a dramatic decrease in intensity of this band using lysates made from the both knock out DRG tissues when compared with wild type control animals (>4 fold decrease of control Figure 5.1). When the density in the control group was standardized to 1.0, the average densities were 0.172 ± 0.08 of ERαKO and 0.262 ± 0.10 of ERβKO in P2X3 receptors, and 0.59 ± 0.06 of ERαKO and 0.391 ± 0.04 of ERβKO in TRPV1 receptors, suggesting that both P2X3 and TRPV1 protein decreased in DRG, $P < 0.05$, $n = 10$.

Nociceptive (small diameter) DRG neurons also express capsaicin-sensitive vanilloid (TRPV1) receptors. TRPV1positive neurons were categorized according to their labeling patterns and were expressed as a percentage of the total number of TRPV1 -positive cells. Immunohistochemical signal from ERαKO, ERβKO and WT mice was measured by computerized image analysis (Figure 5.2). TRPV1 receptor expression and activity might be considered as markers for a specific subtype of sensory neurons, and their activation by exogenous stimuli (e.g., capsaicin) could be a useful tool to exam the possible modulatory effects of pain-related substances.

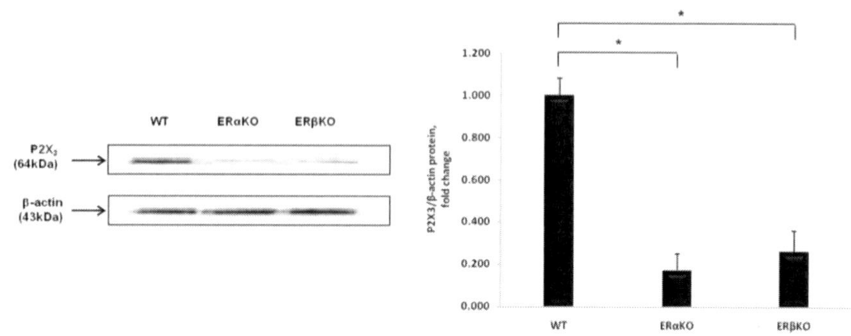

Figure 5.1. Western blot analysis of DRG lysates shows reduced expression of P2X3 and TRPV1 in both knock-out mice.

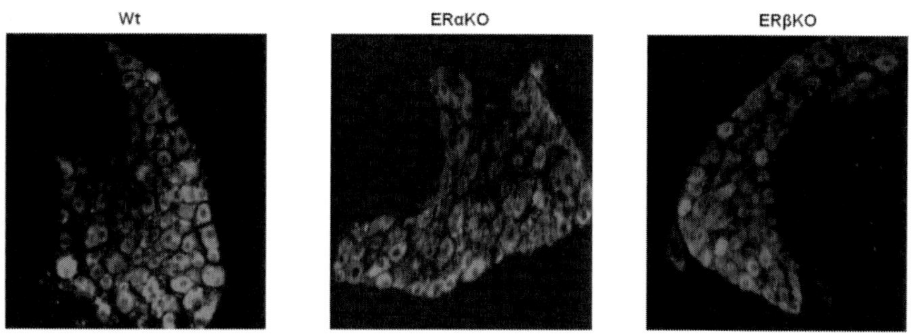

Figure 5.2. Expression of TRPV1 receptors in dorsal root ganglion neurons from Wt, ERαKO, and ERβKO in vivo.

Endometriosis is one of the most common benign gynecological diseases, characterized by the presence of endometrial tissue outside the uterine cavity, most commonly implanted over visceral and peritoneal surfaces within the female pelvis. Clinical studies have shown that it may occur in up to 10-15% of women of reproductive age. Symptoms of endometriosis are usually associated with pelvic pain, including recurrent painful periods, painful intercourse, and painful defecation during menstruation, chronic lower abdominal pain and hypersensitivity. Unfortunately, understanding of the mechanisms of endometriosis-associated pain and its management in women is currently insufficient. Studies have shown possible mechanisms of chronic pelvic pain associated with endometriosis could be due to persistent nociceptive input from endometrial tissues that lead to peripheral and central sensitisation resulting in increased responsiveness of dorsal root ganglion and dorsal horn neurons. Indeed, recent studies in human and animals have shown that peritoneal endometrial lesions are richly innervated by Aδ and C sensory nerve fibers, which positively stained by substance P or calcitonin gene-related peptide. Several lines of evidence indicated that there is a close relationship between nerve fiber density and endometriosis-associated pain. There is a significant increase in nerve fiber density in women with endometriosis who reported pelvic pain, suggesting these nerve fibers may play an important role in the mechanisms of pain generation. Accumulating literatures described that SP presents in the myometrium and is involved in the inflammatory and pain responses, suggesting a possible role of substance P (SP) nerve fibers in the generation of pain related to endometriosis. SP, which is synthesized and contained in 20–30% of DRG neurons, is involved in the transmission of nociceptive information to the central nerve system. SP is contained primarily in, and co-released from, small-diameter primary afferent fibers on noxious stimulation. Activation of nociceptive C and Aδ primary afferent fibers by electrical, chemical, or mechanical stimulation has been reported to release SP. Visceral nociceptive C-fibers can be activated by SP, representing an endogenous system regulating inflammatory, immune responses, and visceral hypersensitivity. SP afferent fibers play an important role in the pathogenesis of visceral hyperalgesia, suggesting critical role of SP in regulation of pelvic nociception associated with endometriosis. ATP is a peripheral mediator of pain which contributes to the activation of sensory afferents by activating ATP receptors following inflammation or nerve injury. It may correlate with SP release and play an important role in modulating nociception in primary sensory neurons. Local injections of ATP and ATP analogs to the rat hindpaw elicit spontaneous pain behaviors, hyperalgesia and allodynia which can be augmented by inflammation, indicating ATP might be involved in visceral hyperalgesia associated with endometriosis. Although these findings reveal the greater abundance of primary sensory nerve fibers clearly present within the peritoneal endometrial lesions in patients diagnosed with endometriosis, and these nerve fibers may play an important role in pain generation associated with endometriosis, pain mechanisms associated with endometriosis are still not well known, and the role of these primary sensory nerve fibers has not been specifically determined.

Our data support the idea that E2 modulates nociceptive responses in pelvic pain syndromes such as endometriosis, however, whether E2 is pro- or anti-nociceptive remains unresolved. Within the context of our hypothesis visceral nociception and nociceptor sensitization appear to be regulated by P2X3 and TRPV1. E2 modulates DRG neurons response to ATP and capsaicin suggesting that visceral afferent nociceptors are modulated by E2 in the DRG. The DRG is an important site of visceral afferent convergence and cross-sensitization. We have demonstrated that 17-β estradiol, the most common form of estrogen act on functional properties of P2X3 and TRPV1 receptors in DRG neurons in vitro. DRG neurons from Wt and knock-out mice responded to P2X3 and TRPV1 activation. We also studied the long-term (chronic) exposure to E2 on sensory neurons that mimics the temporal pattern of circulating E2 levels in cycling female rodents which is equivalent to an E2 primal action on animal reproductive behavior. The localization of ER in DRG neurons strongly suggest that E2 modulates visceral pain processing peripherally. Adult DRG neurons in short-term culture retain the expression of receptors (P2X and TRPV1) which mediate the response to putative nociceptive signals. They continue to respond to ER agonists mimicking in vivo activation. An important advantage is that these neurons can be studied apart from endogenous signals. Our data clearly showed the new role of nociceptors in pathophysiological aspects of chronic pelvic pain and potential way of designing future therapies.

References

Berkley, K. J., A. J. Rapkin, et al. The pains of endometriosis. *Science*, 2005, 308(5728): 1587-1589.

Burnstock, G. Purine-mediated signalling in pain and visceral perception. *Trends Pharmacol Sci*, 2001, 22(4): 182-188.

Chaban, V. V. Visceral sensory neurons that innervate both uterus and colon express nociceptive TRPv1 and P2X3 receptors in rats. *Ethn Dis,* 2008, 18(2 Suppl 2): S2-20-24.

Chaban, V. V. Peripheral sensitization of sensory neurons. *Ethn Dis*, 2010, 20(1 Suppl 1): S1-3-6.

Giamberardino, M. A., R. Costantini, et al. Viscero-visceral hyperalgesia: characterization in different clinical models. *Pain*, 2010, 151(2): 307-322.

Koshimizu, T. A., F. Van Goor, et al. Characterization of calcium signaling by purinergic receptor-channels expressed in excitable cells. *Mol Pharmacol*, 2000, 58(5): 936-945.

Malykhina, A. P. Neural mechanisms of pelvic organ cross-sensitization. *Neuroscience,* 2007, 149(3): 660-672.

Pezzone, M. A., R. Liang, et al. A model of neural cross-talk and irritation in the pelvis: implications for the overlap of chronic pelvic pain disorders. *Gastroenterology,* 2005, 128(7): 1953-.

Chapter 6

Clinical Aspects of Visceral Pain

Abstract

This chapter represents a review of clinical data obtained in hospital setting by validating the new instrument "The Suffering Scale." Suffering Scale may provide a rapid assessment of the affective dimension of pain and can be used as a tool to help to determine whether the patient with chronic pelvic pain (CPP) could benefit from multi-disciplinary pain management. The Suffering Scale may possibly provide more "user friendly" way to explore the CPP. This instrument will help to determine if there are any correlation between CPP diagnostic subtypes, severity of pain, duration of pain, trauma history, various aspects of family history, other pain complaints and psychological history.

Etiology of Chronic Pelvic Pain

One of the presentation of visceral pain Chronic Pelvic Pain (CPP) syndrome is affecting up to 25% of reproductive age patients (about a billion worldwide) and resulting in dysmenorrhea, menstrual irregularities, and reduced fecundity in women and chronic prostatitis as the most common CPP in men. As result of these disorders chronic back pain can develop. In female the most common cause of CPP are endometriosis, vulvodynia/ vestibulodynia and pelvic floor myalgia. Chronic pain adversely affects mood, social and professional life and general well-being. Thus, assessing the impact of the pain on various domains of a patient's existence has become an important focus in the clinical management.

The objective of this study was to assess the internal consistency of the new instrument "The Suffering Scale" in clinical context of the gynecological pelvic pain clinic and compared the Suffering Scale (SS) scores to other validated pain questionnaires instruments: Brief Pain Inventory (BPI), McGill Questionnaire, the Hospital and Depression (HAD) questionnaire, Somatic Symptoms Severity Scale (SSSS) and Coping Strategy Questionnaire (CSQ) for the patients with chronic pelvic pain currently used in clinical practice. We used cross-sectional study of 80 adult patients admitted to the women pelvic pain clinic at University of California, Los Angeles. Data obtained from SS were compared to 5 different validated questionnaires used in the clinics; Brief Pain Inventory (BPI), McGill Questionnaire, the Hospital and Depression (HAD) questionnaire, Somatic Symptoms Severity Scale (SSSS) and Coping Strategy Questionnaire (CSQ). Of the 80 subjects 45% were married or living together, 54% were employed, 58% with college education or higher and 23% with high school education or less. Mean age was of 36.1 + 13.1 years (range 16-80 years) (Chaban et al. 2009)

Principal component analysis extracted three factors in the SS that accounted for 72% of the variance. All the scales used were internally consistent, with values of Cronback's coefficient (alpha) being 0.72 to 0.92. For the SS alpha was satisfactory high (alpha = 0.88). There was significant correlation between the SS and all other instruments. Our data suggests that SS mostly correlates with SCQ, HAD, McGill and BPI. This scale may be an effective clinical tool targeting affective factors that lead maintenance of chronic pain states and may serve to predict whether to limit treatment to pelvic therapy or to refer for multidisciplinary approaches early in the diagnostic and therapeutic process.

CPP defined as pelvic pain in the same location for at least 6 months. Most women with complaints of pelvic pain will undergo laparoscopy to both diagnose and treat these diseases, but laparoscopy is often is unsuccessful due to lack of intraperitoneal pathology or altered pain processing. Pain out of proportion to identifiable pathology is the most immediate and dramatic consequence of disorders associated with CPP and is responsible for a highly negative impact on quality of life and substantial workforce loss. Due to the alarming situation and unmet need, the USA and other countries have launched a call for more focused research on improving the diagnosis and treatment of CPP syndrome.

Pain is subjective feeling and thus difficult to be standardized and parameterized in a mathematical fashion for scientific analysis. Often the etiology of CPP is not clear, as there are many symptoms of the reproductive system, gastrointestinal and urinary tracts, musculoskeletal, neurological and psychological systems that often co-occur in the same patient. The variation of pain symptoms and pain perception and behavioral responses to pain in these patients is poorly understood. There is often no clear relationship between the severity of the chronic pelvic pain and pathology in the pelvic viscera, including reproductive tract (ovaries and uterus), urinary bladder, and colon. Studies of the sympathetic nervous system in individuals with CPP associated with gynecological diseases, painful bladder syndrome/ interstitial cystitis (PBS) and functional bowel disorders such as IBS suggest a model in which alteration in the central stress circuits in predisposed individuals may be triggered by and then maintain the pain and pathophysiological changes in the viscera. CPP patients have significantly more depression, psychological and somatic complains and more often give a history of physical, sexual or emotional abuse or trauma. Chronic pain adversely affects mood, social, and professional life and general well-being. These quality of life issues can affect severity of pain, degree of impairment resulting from a painful condition and success of pain treatment modalities in alleviating pain. A consideration of pain mechanisms must also include the neural systems modulating pain, for it is well known that pain can be profoundly influenced by other somatic stimuli and by attentional, emotional, and cognitive factors. The history and physical examination are crucial in evaluating a suffering patient and must address all of the possible systems potentially involved in chronic pelvic pain, not just the reproductive system.

Pain is a complex and individual experience that is often difficult for patients to fully describe using a conventional pain intensity scale (Melzack 2008). Health-related quality of life encompasses those aspects of health and well-being valued by patients, specifically, their physical, emotional, and cognitive function, and their ability to participate in meaningful activities within their family, workplace, and community. Up to date the evaluation and treatment of chronic pain now incorporates a Visual Analog Pain Scale (0-10) for the assessment of pain severity. The visual analogue scale has been widely used for pain assessment in pain clinics and has been described in the literature in detail (Parazzini, Ricci et al. 2001). Nevertheless, the extent and impact of the pain associated with CPP and associated gynecological manifestations does not seem to be readily assessed with available instruments. There are also many questionnaires which have been developed to assess quality of life, depression and anxiety; and some of these have been used in the multidisciplinary assessment of patients with CPP.

There is concern that not enough emphasis is placed on clinical face validity (i.e., issues which are important to patients and reflect their experiences and concerns). Systematic review of published studies indicated that the SF-36 was used most frequently by being employed in 53% of the studies (Neelakantan et al. 2004) Overall, quality assessment showed that only 22% of these studies met more than half of the criteria for face validity. Among existing instruments, compliance with the quality criteria for measurement properties was higher than for clinical face validity. There is a need to develop disease specific quality of life instruments for CPP. There is need for more "user friendly" way to explore the effects of CPP on quality of life and can be extensively used in clinical practice as additional diagnostic tool. Future studies can therefore determine if new instruments for determining quality of life can help to guide general medical and gynecologic physicians in diagnosis of CPP syndrome and in choosing a multiplatform, multidisciplinary management approach. CPP syndrome implies the pain symptoms are not just a manifestation of a peripheral pelvic abnormality, but a complex entity in which traditional gynecologic therapy is less effective due to altered central nervous system processing of pain signals.

In previous study author of this book conducted a survey of female patients attending two Pain Clinics in Los Angeles, USA with full range of gynecological disorders (see Table 6.1) seen in referral practice. All English-speaking patients between 16 and 80 years old were asked to fill out a Pain Assessment Form which is a comprehensive form of the health outcome of the current study. Completed responses of the total 80 participants were analyzed. All predicted variables were assessed at baseline. Patients were asked for their date of birth, year of formal education. Of the 80 subjects 45% were married or living together, 54% employed, 58% with college education or higher and 23% with high school education or less. Mean age was of 36.13 + 13.1 years (range 16-80 years) (Table 6.1)

Internal Consistency

Internal consistency of the suffering scale, as calculated by Cronbach's coefficient alpha, should be at least 0.60 for a self-report instrument to be reliable and at least 0.80 when used as a screening instrument.

Table 6.1. Population characteristics (n=80)

Variable	Number (%)
Demographics	
Age, years	
16-25	14
25-35	38
35-45	14
45-55	15
>55	19
Education	
College and higher	58
Employment	
Employed	60
Unemployed	33
Physical Activity	
Exercising regularly	62
Not exercising	38
Personal Habit	
Alcohol consumption	4
Smoking	7
Caffeinated drinks	14

Table 6.2. Study Sample Diagnoses

DIAGNOSES (Groups)	Number	%
1. Endometriosis or adenomyosis	15	19
2. Myofascial abdominal wall or pelvic floor tension myalgia or abdominal wall neuropathy	26	33
3. Vulvodynia or vestibulodynia or pudendal neuropathy	39	48

Several studies conclude that the valid scale fulfils these criteria when Cronbach's alpha has been found to be 0.78-0.93 (Stordal, Nygaard et al. 2001). The stability of the findings on the internal consistency of the quality of life instrument/scale supports the robustness of the scale as a screening instrument. In our study we measured the internal consistency of different instruments with Cronbach's coefficient (alpha). Our data indicated that all instruments used in this study were satisfactory (standardized alpha had values of 0.73 to 0.92) and the Cronbach's alpha value is satisfactory high (value = 0.88) for the Suffering Scale (Table 6.3). We performed factor analysis using the principal component analysis (PCA) with the number of factors defined by eigenvalues = >1.

Table 6.3. Internal Consistency of the Scales

Scale	# of items		Reliability
	Alpha		Standardized alpha
SS	10	0.88	0.88
BPI	10	0.22	0.92
MCGILL	18	0.87	0.87
HAD	14	0.83	0.84
SSSS	15	0.76	0.77
CSQ	8	0.74	0.73

SS- Suffering Scale.
BPI- Brief Pain Questionnaire.
MCGILL- McGill Short Questionnaire.
HAD- Hospital and Depression Rating Scale.
SSSS- Somatic Symptom Severity Scale.
CSQ- Coping Strategy Questionnaire.

Table 6.4. Factor Analysis (PCA) of the Suffering Scale Components

Question	Factor 1	Factor 2	Factor 3
SS1	752	409	-080
SS2	611	490	-017
SS3	259	593	561
SS4	404	138	-778
SS5	782	236	-100
SS6	715	-332	131
SS7	727	-504	093
SS8	868	-104	014
SS9	798	-312	231
SS10	797	-073	-050
Eigen value	3.57	2.19	1.41
Explained variance	35.72	21.88	14.14

The analysis revealed three factors. The three factors for the suffering scale were related to the following pain dimensions: hopelessness/ helplessness, social support, and sexuality. The factor 1 includes the following modalities: future planning and goal setting, grieving for former self, isolation, helplessness and hopelessness; factor 2 includes questions about personal and professional happiness and anhedonia. As a separate factor 3 is a pain score (Table 6.4). The eigenvalues for the rotated three factors were 3.57, 2.19, and 1.41respectively. The three factors explained 71.8% of the total variance.

Correlational Analyses among the Suffering Scale and Other Validated Instruments

For the correlation analysis between the Suffering Scale and other validated instruments in the study we developed and used an algorithm of scoring. Correlation coefficients between the scores were used. Please, note that HAD scale was scored for 2 subscales: HAD I- anxiety and HAD II-depression. BPI also was scored separately for BPI I- pain severity subscale and BPI II- pain interference subscale. There was significant correlation between the Suffering Scale (SS) and all other instruments. Our data suggests that SS mostly correlates with SCQ, HAD II, McGill and BPI I with Pearson correlation values (all significant at $p < 0.001$ in 2-tailed tests) (Table 6.5).

Table 6.5. Pearson Correlation Score between the Suffering Scale and Other Scales

Instrument	SS Score
BPI I	0.454
BPI II	0.404
HAD I	0.551
HAD II	0.703
McGill	0.465
SSSS	0.390
CSQ	0.676

We determined if there were any correlations among pain diagnosis and different instruments. The Suffering Scale (SS) score is relatively higher than any other instrument however we did not find any specificity between three different groups of diagnoses for any of the validated scales used in this study. Multiple analyses were conducted to determine the reliability of new instrument- the Suffering Scale (SS), the relation between the SS factors and measures of relationship of SS to other validated instruments. The items in the SS questionnaire include a pain score, score for effect of pain on sexual/sensual life happiness, loss of pleasure with daily activities, future planning and goal setting, isolation, helplessness, and hopelessness: all dimensions that significantly affect "suffering" and pain management. Differences in the severity of pain and pain suffering exist for a broad range of pelvic pain conditions. With this study we hope to confirm the specific impact of factors indicated in the Suffering scale on the quality of life of patients suffering with chronic pelvic pain.

We found that total scores and individual items of all tested instruments- Brief Pain Inventory (BPI I for severity and BPI II for interference), the Hospital and Depression (HAD) rating scale (for anxiety (HAD I) and for depression (HAD II), short-form McGill Pain Questionnaire, Somatic Symptom Severity Scale (SSSS) and Coping Strategy Questionnaire (CSQ) correlate well with the Suffering Scale items and the pain scores. Our data suggest that SS (Cronbach's coefficient equal 0.88, Table 3) is very reliable and precise instrument which will guide physician in their therapeutic intervention criteria. The pain scores, sexual /sensual life happiness, anhedonia, future planning and goal setting, isolation, helplessness, and hopelessness are all significantly affect pain management. Thus, from a public health prospective, the outcome of this study can have a substantial impact on our knowledge of pain-related diseases and may help to achieve a deeper understanding the mechanisms of pain-associated symptoms. Only a thorough understanding of the mechanism implicated in the phenomenon of pain can truly contribute to the designing of new and more efficient therapies for chronic pelvic pain. Our data suggest that SS mostly correlated with HAD II and CSQ (Pearson correlations are 0.703 and 0.676 respectively, Table 6.5).

Even we did not anticipate using SS as diagnostic tool but rather than quality of life instrument, we found that overall SS scored better in all three groups of diagnoses than other instruments (Table 6.6). Differences between the patients in pain tolerance exist in the prevalence and severity of a broad range of diseases, disorders and conditions. In calling for greater focus on pain-based biomedical research, clinical community may identify barriers to the achievement of knowledge about these diseases-including ethical, sociological and scientific factors.

Table 6.6. Means Scores for 3 Groups of the Diagnoses

Instrument	Mean (+SD)		
	Group I	Group II	Group III
SS	43.07+20.7	49.04+18.5	49.6+19.8
BPI I	6.6+4.1	8.6+3.1	6.8+3.1
BPI II	24.5+11.3	32.7+9.2	29.4+8.9
McGill	17.2+8.3	21.6+10.7	21.3+9.4
HAD I	8.7+4.2	10.07+3.9	9.8+3.9
HAD II	4.7+2.9	5.6+3.6	6.2+4.7
SSSS	10.1+4.1	11.6+6.1	9.2+4.3
CSQ	13.7+7.1	18.2+9.1	14.9+8.2

SS- Suffering Scale.
BPI I- severity subscale of Brief Pain Inventory.
BPI II- interference subscale of Brief Pain Inventory.
HAD I- anxiety subscale of Hospital and Depression Rating Scale.
HAD II- depression subscale of Hospital and Depression Rating Scale.
MCGILL- McGill Short Questionnaire.
SSSS- Somatic Symptom Severity Scale.
CSQ- Coping Strategy Questionnaire.

Therefore, this study provides new information that certain coping strategies may have significant effect on treatment of many disorders associated with chronic pelvic pain. One of these disorders is endometriosis which is an estrogen-dependent disorder, defined as the presence of endometrial tissue outside of the uterus in lesions of varying sizes and appearance containing endometrial glands and stroma. It may be asymptomatic or associated with symptoms of pain and/or infertility. It is found on the peritoneum and ovaries, in the rectovaginal septum, and in other sites within and outside the pelvis. Data provided following the 10th World Congress on Endometriosis held in Melbourne suggest that endometriosis affects an estimated 1 in 10 women in the reproductive-age group.

This prevalence increases up to 30% in women with infertility and to 50% in infertile women with a normal cycle whose partner has normal reproductive system. Although it is difficult to generate accurate figures for costs associated with endometriosis, recent studies have estimated an annual cost for endometriosis in the United States at $18.8 and $22 billion when direct treatment costs and indirect costs such as lost work productivity are combined.

Although the existence of endometriosis has been known for more than 100 years, our current knowledge of its pathogenesis, the spontaneous evolution of the disease, and the pathophysiology of the related infertility and chronic pelvic pain, remain unclear. One of the major issues identified as impacting on the capacity to undertake endometriosis research is the need for multidisciplinary expertise. There is a need for a multidisciplinary approach to research in all aspects of endometriosis, to include reproductive medicine physicians, epidemiologists, pain specialists, biostatisticians, bioinformaticians, and others to enable effective, accurate, and timely diagnosis, determination of those at risk, and multidisciplinary therapeutic approaches. The Suffering Scale validated in this study is a great example of a new dimension in the multidisciplinary treatment of endometriosis and associated with this disease chronic pelvic pain syndrome.

Vulvodynia is a problem most family physicians can expect to encounter. It is a syndrome of unexplained vulvar pain, frequently accompanied by physical disabilities, limitation of daily activities, sexual dysfunction and psychologic distress. The patient's vulvar pain usually has an acute onset and, in most cases, becomes a chronic problem lasting months to years. The pain is often described as burning or stinging, or a feeling of rawness or irritation. Vulvodynia may have multiple causes, with several subsets, including cyclic vulvovaginitis, vulvar vestibulitis syndrome, essential (dysesthetic) vulvodynia and vulvar dermatoses. Evaluation should include a thorough history and physical examination Proper treatment mandates that the correct type of vulvodynia be identified. Depending on the specific diagnosis, treatment may include besides anti-pain medications antidepressants, physical therapy with biofeedback and psychotherapy. Since vulvodynia is often a chronic condition, regular medical follow-up and referral to a support group are helpful for most patients. We hope that outcome from this study will help physicians to refer patients to appropriate therapy based on their score using the Suffering Scale.

Although many pain-associated functional somatic syndromes such as irritable bowel syndrome, interstitial cystitis, fibromyalgia show substantial overlap with gynecological disorders described in our project such as endometriosis, vulvodynia and myofascial abdominal wall or pelvic floor tension myalgia, treatment research is mostly confined to single syndromes, with a lack of valid and generally accepted diagnostic criteria across medical specialties. Non-pharmacological treatments involving active participation of patients, such as psychotherapy, seem to be more effective than those that involve passive physical measures, including injections and operations. Pharmacological agents with CNS action seem to be more consistently effective than drugs aiming at restoration of peripheral physiological dysfunction.

A balance between biomedical, organ-oriented, and cognitive interpersonal approaches is most appropriate at this truly psychosomatic interface. In view of the iatrogenic component in the maintenance of functional somatic syndromes, doctor-centered interventions and close observation of the doctor–patient relationship are of particular importance. From this prospective, the Suffering Scale as new instrument to assess patient's quality of life may have significant beneficial effect on therapeutic intervention for patients with CPP and functional disorders. Future evaluation in general and pelvic pain specifically will incorporate the

References

Chaban V., M. Shaheen, A. Rapkin Suffering Scale- a Novel Way to Assess Pain and Suffering in Patients with Chronic Pelvic Pain. *Annals of Epidemiology* 2009 19(9): 675-676.

Melzak R. The future of pain. Nature Reviews Drug Discovery, 2008, 7: 629.

Neelakantan, D., F. Omojole, et al. Quality of life instruments in studies of chronic pelvic pain: a systematic review. *J Obstet Gynaecol*, 2004, 24(8): 851-8.

Parazzini, F., E. Ricci, et al. Risk of endometrial cancer after use of fertility drugs. *Hum Reprod,* 2001, 16(1): 196.

Stordal, K., E. A. Nygaard, et al. Organic abnormalities in recurrent abdominal pain in children. *Acta Paediatr*, 2001, 90(6): 638-42.

Chapter 7

Visceral Pain: Time for a Paradigm Shift

Abstract

This chapter describes new factors for visceral pain. Role of visceral and somatic nociceptors discussed in details. Patients with chronic pelvic pain (CPP) frequently have pain from several pelvic organs. The most common diagnoses include endometriosis, interstitial cystitis/ Painful Bladder Syndrome (PBS), Irritable Bowel Syndrome (IBS), pelvic floor tension myalgia, vulvar vestibulitis and vulvodynia. IBS and pelvic floor tension myalgia and neuropathy may have no clearly demonstrable pathologic tissue changes. Most diagnoses associated with chronic pelvic pain have a high rate of recurrence and all are considered to be chronic conditions with a relapsing course. Despite a successful reduction of pain using currently available treatments, visceral pain returns in majority of patients. Often the etiology of visceral pain is not clear, as there are many symptoms of the reproductive system, gastrointestinal and urinary tracts, musculoskeletal, neurological and psychological systems that often co-occur in the same patient. It is a time for paradigm shift in our understanding of nociceptive mechanisms of visceral pain.

The Dorsal Root Ganglion in Visceral Pain As a Target for Neuromodulation

There is no shortage of opportunities for clinical research in developing potentially highly successful anti-nociceptive therapies. The reader may find additional targets of opportunity in the literature of other nociceptive disorders that follow the dictum of the momentum that treatment success seems to be inversely proportional to the molecular understanding of the etiology and pathophysiology.. The treating clinician is often tempted to take a unidimensional approach and focus on one organ system and ignore the psychological and behavioral manifestations of the chronic pain. A major aim of this book is to challenge the traditional concept of a multitude of unrelated, individual pain experiences, which are the "property" of different medical subspecialties, and for which different therapies are developed. Experts generally agree that in women are more likely affected by visceral pain conditions, including IC/PBS, IBS and CPP.

Infection or injury to a particular organ or body part could initiate a period of enhanced nociceptive processing, associated with peripheral and central sensitization. While such sensitization is generally self-limited and counter-regulated by endogenous pain inhibition systems in the majority of patients, in a patient with vulnerability factors for chronic visceral pain (alterations in attentional or affective modulation of nociceptive signals and compromised endogenous pain inhibition systems), such peripherally triggered symptoms could develop into a chronic pain syndrome.

Number of molecules and neurotrophic factors are involved in hyperalgesia and overall sensory neuron sensitization (Jankowski and Koerber, 2010).The inflammatory process produces mediators which activate nociceptors by interacting with ligand-gated ion channels or by sensitizing primary afferents (Dai et al. 2004). One mechanism for sensitization involves phosphorylation of ion channels and receptors including P2X3 and TRPV1 receptors. One mechanism for sensitization involves phosphorylation of ion channels and receptors including P2X3 and TRPV1 receptors. Inflammation does not change the percentage of total cells responding to ATP but sensitizes the ATP response by increasing the expression of P2X3. Thus, the greater behavioral sensitivity during the inflammation is due to a twofold to threefold increase in ATP responses suggesting that a small amount of ATP would evoke depolarization sufficient to elicit action potentials in DRG neurons (Xu and Huang 2002). Furthermore, inflamed tissues augment nociceptor responsiveness by acting on TRPV1 (Negri et al. 2006). Gastrointestinal inflammation modulates the intrinsic properties of nociceptive dorsal root ganglia neurones, which innervate the GI tract and these changes are important in the genesis of abdominal pain and visceral hyperalgesia. Neurons exhibit hyperexcitability characterized by a decreased threshold for activation and increased firing rate (Beyak and Vanner 2005). Inflammation upregulates the activity of NMDARs in all DRG neurons within ganglia innervating viscera. Inflammation upregulates the activity of NMDARs in all DRG neurons within ganglia innervating viscera (Li et al. 2006). Sensitization may also account for a lowered nociceptive threshold to mechanical manipulation of the inflamed area. Within the context of our cross-sensitization hypothesis, inflammation sensitizes non-inflamed viscera that are innervated by the same DRG and/or cross-sensitization occurs as a result of intra-DRG release of sensitizing mediators such as ATP within the DRG. A large body of literature supports the idea that E2 modulates nociceptive responses in pelvic and other visceral pain syndromes; however, this mechanism remains unresolved. The DRG is an important site of visceral afferent convergence and cross-sensitization.

Estradiol Inhibits TRPV1 Receptors Activation by Capsaicin in Visceral DRG Neurons

Emerging evidence support a role of the transient receptor potential subfamily 1 (TRPV1) receptors in modulating nociceptive signaling at the level of primary sensory neurons. Our data showed that lumbosacral DRG neurons (L1-S1) express capsaicin-sensitive TRPV1, and both ERα and ERβ receptors. In this study we demonstrated the expression of TRPV1 receptors by Western blotting and immunohistochemistry and the effect of 17β-estradiol (E2β) on capsaicin-induced $[Ca^{2+}]_i$ increase in DRG neurons collected from wild type (Wt), estrogen receptor-α knock out (ERαKO) and estrogen receptor-β knock out (ERβKO) mice. Our data indicated a significant decrease for TRPV1 in ERαKO (all levels) and ERβKO (mostly observed in L1, L2, and S1). In the contest to visceral pain, the transient receptor potential subfamily 1 (TRPV1) receptor is a sensory neuron-specific cation channel and plays an important role in a ligand-gated ion channel that integrates multiple pain transmission including vanilloids, protons, inflammation induced thermal hyperalgesia (Caterina et al. 2000; Davis et al. 2000). Peripheral sensitization can develop in response to sustain stimulation, inflammation, and nerve injury. Visceral pain is different from cutaneous pain based on clinical, neurophysiological and pharmacological characteristics.

The expression of TRPV1 receptor is widespread in several areas of the nervous system, but it is particularly strong in dorsal root ganglion (DRG) nociceptors. Primary DRG neurons culture have been a useful model system for investigating sensory physiology and putative nociceptive signaling (Chaban et al. 2001). The capsaicin-sensitive primary afferent neurons of small- and medium-diameter neurons mediate nociceptive-like behaviors suggesting that TRPV1 expressing neurons are nociceptors. Evidence for TRPV1's role in there pathogenesis in the transmission of selective nociception modalities comes from studies showing that mice lacking TRP1R gene have deficits in thermal- or inflammatory-induced hyperalgesia (Davis et al. 2000). It is strongly attenuated and the response of primary sensory neurons to the same stimuli is severely impaired (Caterina et al. 2000). Activation of TRPV1 receptors results in the production of a cation current with a subsequent depolarization and opening of voltage-gated Ca^{2+} channels (VGCC) (Koshimizu et al. 2000). A sensation of pain is produced by depolarization of the peripheral nerve terminals (Waxman et al. 2000).

Capsaicin-induced TPRV1 receptor-mediated changes in $[Ca^{2+}]_i$ may represent a level of DRG activation to noxious cutaneous stimulation while ATP-induced changes in $[Ca^{2+}]_i$ may reflect the level of DRG neuron sensitization to noxious visceral stimuli since ATP is released by noxious stimuli and tissue damage near the primary afferent nerve terminals (Burnstock 2001). In the view of this fact, TRPV1 receptor expression and activity might be considered as markers for a specific subtype of sensory neurons, and their activation by exogenous stimuli (e.g., capsaicin) could be a useful tool to exam the possible modulatory effects of pain-related substances. Our study showed that the expression of nociceptive transient (TRPV1) receptor in DRG neurons significantly decreased in sensory neurons from ERαKO and ERβKO mice and find a novel pathway that 17β-estradiol, acting at the level of the plasma membrane, attenuates capsaicin-induced $[Ca^{2+}]i$ fluxes. The rapid estradiol attenuation of capsaicin-induced $[Ca^{2+}]_i$ fluxes in DRG neurons suggests that 17β-estradiol may alter nociceptive transmission at the primary afferent level. We demonstrate the role of estrogen knock out- α and -β in the context of the influence of capsaicin-induced TPRV1 receptor-mediated changes in $[Ca^{2+}]_i$ increase.

In that study, we have used 6~8 weeks old female wild type (Wt, C57Bl6J), ERαKO (B6.129P2-Esr1tm1Ksk/J), and ERβKO (B6.129P2-

Esr2tm1Unc/J) mice (Jackson Laboratory, Bar Harbor, ME). Upon arrival mice were housed in microisolator caging and maintained on a 12-h light/dark cycle in a temperature-controlled environment with access to food and water ad libitum for two weeks. In some experiments we used animals from a breeding colony. Age-matched (8–10 wks old) heterozygous mutant mice lacking the gene male (ERα−/−) and female (ERα−/−) for ERα (ERα−/−), and the deficiency ERβ (ERβ−/−) mice were bred into heterozygous mutant female mice (ERβ−/−) and homozygous male mutant mice (ERβ−/−). The isolation procedure and primary culture of mouse lumbosacral DRG has been published in detail (Chaban et al. 2003). DRG tissues were obtained from C57Bl6J (30g), ERαKO and ERβKO (Taconic; 20 g) transgenic types. Briefly, lumbosacral adult DRGs (level L1-S1) were collected under sterile technique and placed in ice-cold medium Dulbecco's Modified Eagle's Medium (DMEM; Sigma-Aldrich St. Louis, MO). Adhering fat and connective tissue were removed and each DRG was minced with scissors and placed immediately in a medium consisting of 5 ml of DMEM containing 0.5 mg/ml of trypsin (Sigma, type III), 1 mg/ml of collagenase (Sigma, type IA) and 0.1 mg/ml of DNAase (Sigma, type III) and kept at 37°C for 30 minutes with agitation. After dissociation of the cell ganglia, soybean trypsin inhibitor (Sigma, type III) was used to terminate cell dissociation. Cell suspensions were centrifuged for one minute at 1000 rpm and the cell pellet were resuspended in DMEM supplemented with 5% fetal bovine serum, 2 mM glutamine-penicillin-streptomycin mixture, 1 μg/ml DNAase and 5 ng/ml NGF (Sigma). Cells were placed on Matrigel® (Invitrogen, Carlsbad, CA) coated 15-mm coverslips (Collaborative Research Co., Bedford, PA) and kept at 37°C in 5% CO_2 incubator for 24 hours, given fresh media and maintained in primary culture until used for experimental procedures.

The expressions of TRPV1 receptors in L1-S1 DRGs were studied by using Western blot analyses. Tissues from Wt (C57Bl6J), ERαKO, and ERβKO mice were quick frozen in tubes on dry ice during collection. L1-S1 DRG were combined, homogenized by mechanical disruption on ice-cold RIPA buffer plus protease inhibitors and incubated on ice for 30 minutes. Homogenates were then spun at 5000 g for 15 minutes and supernatants collected. Total protein was determined on the supernatants using the BCA microtiter method (Pierce, Rockford, IL, USA). Samples containing equal amounts of protein (40 μg) were electrophoresed under denaturing conditions using Novex Mini-cell system (San Diego, CA, USA) and reagents (NuPage 4 ~ 12% Bis-Tris gel and MOPS running buffer). After electrophoretic transfer onto nitrocellulose membrane using the same system, the membrane was blocked with 5% non-fat dry milk (NFDM) in 25 mM TRIS buffered saline, pH 7.2, plus Tween 20 (TBST) for 1 hour at room temperature, followed by incubation with polyclonal rabbit antibody against TRPV1 receptor (1:1000, Neuromics, Edina, MN) for overnight at 4oC. The membrane was then washed in TBST plus NFDM, and incubated with secondary antibody, HRP conjugated and rabbit IgG (Santa Cruz Biotechnology, CA) at 1:5000 in the same buffer for 2 hours at room temperature. Following a final wash in TBST without NFDM, the membrane was incubated with ECL+ (Amersham, Arlington Heights, Ill., USA) substrate for HRP. Membranes were probed with primary antibody and corresponding secondary antibodies, signals were scanned and quantified by Image J version 1.28U and NIH Image 1.60 scan software. Following enhanced chemiluminescence detection of proteins, the membranes were stripped and re-hybridized with β-actin antibody as a loading control. At least three independent cell preparations were used.

For tissue collection DRG from bilateral spinal levels L1-S2 were removed and fixed in 4% paraformaldehyde for overnight at 4oC. DRGs were rinsed in Delbecco's Phosphate Buffered Saline (DPBS) and kept in sucrose (20%, 4°C) for cryoprotection (48 hrs), after which excess liquid was removed. Each DRG was mounted in Tissue-Tek® OCT embedding medium (Sakura Finetek, Torrance, CA), and sectioned at -20oC in a MICROM H505E (Viocompare, San Francisco, CA) cryostat. Sections were cut at 20 μm and collected in PBS. Endogenous tissue peroxidase activity was quenched by soaking the sections for 10 minutes in 3% hydrogen peroxide solution in 0.01 M PBS. The specimens were washed and then treated for 60 minutes in blocking solution, 0.01 M PBS containing 0.5% Triton X-100 and 1% normal donkey serum (NDS) at room temperature. They were processed with TRPV1 receptor antibody (1:5000, Neuromics, Edina, MN) for overnight at 4oC, washed in 0.01 M phosphate-buffered saline (PBS) and 0.01 M Tris Buffered Saline (TBS), followed by incubation in solutions of donkey anti-rabbit fluorophore-conjugated secondary antibodies (1:200, Invitrogen) in 0.01 M Tris Buffered Saline (TBS) for 3 hrs at room temperature. Cells showing no apparent or only faint membrane / intracellular labeling were considered to be negative for TRPV1. TRPV1-positive neurons showed diffuse membrane intracellular labeling were mounted and coverslipped with Aqua Poly Mount (Polisciences, Warrington, PA). Images from at least three sections in each level were taken using Leica DMLB M130X microscope. The total numbers of DRG neurons expressing TRPV1 were counted. Immunohistochemical signal percent was measured by computerized image analysis (Image Pro-Plus, Media Cybernetics, Silver Spring, MD, USA).

Ca^{2+} fluorescence imaging was carried out as previously described (Chaban et al. 2001, Chaban 2010). DRG neurons were loaded with fluorescent dye Fura-2AM (Invitrogen, Carlsbad, CA) for 45 minutes at 37°C in HBSS supplemented with 20 mM HEPES, pH 7.4. The coverslips were mounted on a fast-perfusion chamber P-4 (World Precision Instrument, Sarasota, FL) and placed on a stage of Olympus IX51 inverted microscope (Olympus America, Center Valley, PA). Observations were made at room temperature (20 ~ 25°C) with 20X UApo/340 objective. A fast superfusion system was used to perfuse the cells with perfusion media, estradiol and other chemicals. Fluorescence intensity at 505 nm with excitation at 334 nm and 380 nm were captured as digital images (sampling rates of 0.1-2 s). Regions of interest were identified within the soma from which quantitative measurements were made by re-analysis of stored image sequences using Slidebook® Digital Microscopy software. $[Ca^{2+]}i$ was determined by ratiometric method of Fura-2 fluorescence from calibration of series of buffered Ca^{2+} standards. E2β was applied acutely onto the experimental chamber. Repeated application of drugs was achieved by superfusion in a rapid mixing chamber into individual neurons for specific intervals (100-500 ms). Cells were perfused with experimental media (2 ml/min) using a Rainin® peristaltic pump. The amplitude of $[Ca^{2+}]_i$ response represents the difference between baseline concentration and the transient peak response to drug stimulation. Significant differences in response to chemical stimulation were obtained by comparing $[Ca^{2+}]_i$ increases during the first stimulation with the second. A cell were judged responsive if E2β inhibited the second $[Ca^{2+}]_i$ transient by >30% of the first. This criterion was empirically derived in previous experiments. Statistical analysis was performed using Statistical Package for the Social Sciences 15.0 (SPSS, Chicago, IL, USA). To assess the significance among different groups, data were analyzed with one-way ANOVA followed by Schéffe post hoc test. A $p < 0.05$ was considered statistically significant.

We tested TRPV1 receptors expression by western blot analysis of lysates from wild type, ERαKO, and ERβKO DRG tissues using a TRPV1 specific primary antiserum (Figure 7.1 (a)). An intense band representing a ~130 kDa (TRPV1) was seen in DRG lysates from wild type animals. There was a dramatic decrease in intensity of this band using lysates made from the both knock out DRG tissues when compared with wild type control animals (>2 ~ 3 fold decrease of control Figure 7.1 (b)). The average intensities of the bands in both knock-out mice has statistically significant. When the density in the control group was standardized to 1.0, the average densities were 0.59 ± 0.06

of ERαKO and 0.391 ± 0.04 of ERβKO in TRPV1 receptors, suggesting that TRPV1 protein decreased in DRG, $P < 0.05$, $n = 3$.

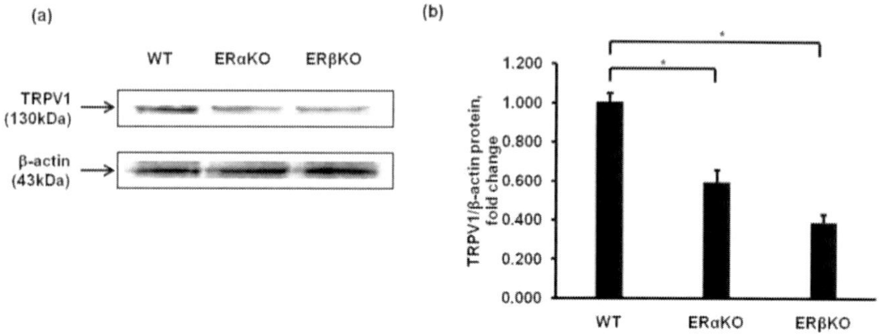

Figure 7.1. Western blot analysis of DRG lysates shows reduced expression of TRPV1 in both knock-out mice. Equal amounts of lysates (40μg) generated from ERαKO and ERβKO DRG neurons, as well as from wild type mice, were electrophoresed under denaturing conditions and probed with a anti-TRPV1 antibodies (n = 3 per group). Representative results with TRPV1 are shown in (a). (b) Both DRG neurons of knock-out mice show a significant reduction in band intensity, 2~3 fold changes of knock-out compared with neurons from wild type (control) DRG. Immunoreactivity is shown as a fold change of the mean value from wild type animals. Quantification of signals from western blots shows statistically significant difference between the intensity of the bands from both knock-out DRG neurons when compared with wild type animals. Values are expressed as mean ± SEM $P < 0.05$, $n = 3$. * indicate significant difference from control.

Our study showed that nociceptive capsaicin-sensitive TRPV1 receptors express in DRG neurons. DRGs section were immunostained with primary antibodies against TRPV1. Neuronal profiles from each four mouse with ERαKO, ERβKO as well as wild type mice were quantified for each fluorescent probe. The TRPV1 receptors are present in DRG neurons. The distributions of labeled dorsal root ganglion neurons represent the statistically significant difference between L1, L2, S1 levels of TRPV1 receptors in both ERαKO and ERβKO DRG neurons when compared with wild type mice. And also there was statistically significant difference L3 and L4 of TRPV1 in wild type compared to ERαKO (Figure 7.2; $P < 0.05$, $n = 4$ per group). To confirm that the capsaicin, a TRPV1 agonist, used in our Ca^{2+} imaging system functional, we applied 100 nM of capsaicin on the DRG cells. The extracellular capsaicin apparently caused $[Ca^{2+}]_i$ increases, which were almost completely blocked by 300 nM capsazepine (CPZ), a TRPV1-selective antagonist.

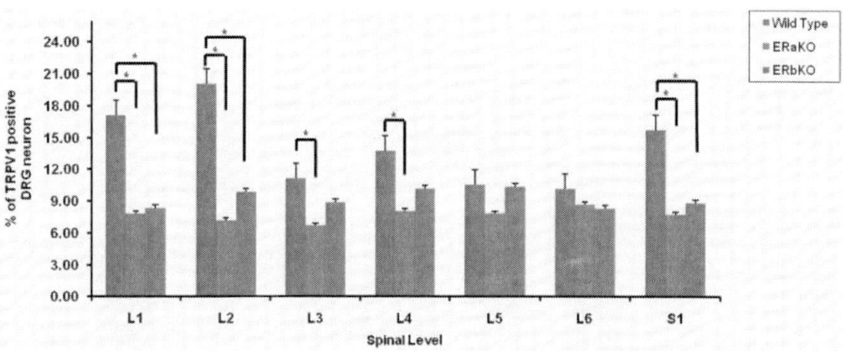

Figure 7.2. Percentage distribution of labeled DRG neurons in ERαKO and ERβKO as well as wild type mice with TRPV1 through lumbar spine level 1 through sacral spine level 1. There was some statistically significant difference between the intensity from knock-out DRG neurons when compared with wild type animals. Values are expressed as mean ± SEM $P < 0.05$, $n = 4$ per group. * indicate significant difference from control.

Brief application of capsaicin (100 nM) by fast superfusion produced $[Ca^{2+}]_i$ spikes. After 10 min washout with HBSS, addtitonal stimulation with capsaicin (100 nM) induced a subsequent $[Ca2+]_i$ fluxes that were similar to the previous stimuli. The estradiol by itself had no effect on basal $[Ca^{2+}]_i$, but 17β-estradiol (100 nM) attenuated the peak of capsaicin-induced $[[Ca^{2+}]_i$ transients. The superfusion with capsaicin (100 nM) induced $[Ca^{2+}]_i$ increase, but this effect was attenuated by 17β-estradiol. We found statistically significant difference in the effect of TRPV1 in wild type mice. This study indicate that the effect of E2β on TRPV1 might be one of the mechanisms for the sensitization of neurons to pain signals and find the mechanism of E2β-mediated changes of TRPV1 activity. E2β (100 nM) by itself had no effect on basal $[Ca^{2+}]_i$ transients, but this hormone attenuated the capsaicin-induced $[Ca^{2+}]_i$ transients in a dose-dependent manner. The effect of estradiol was reversible. The estrogen receptor antagonist ICI 182,780 (1 μM) blocked the 17β-estradiol effect on attenuated capsaicin-induced $[Ca^{2+}]_i$ transients. Besides the Ca^{2+} influx through the membrane, various intracellular Ca^{2+} stores can release and uptake Ca^{2+} to regulate $[Ca^{2+}]_i$. (Figure 7.3).

It has been shown that activation of TRPV1 caused Ca^{2+} influx and release from intracellular stores (Eun et al. 2001). To verify the dependence on Ca^{2+} influx and release from intracellular stores the experiments was conducted in the presence of BAPTA (10 mM), the Ca^{2+} chelator, prior to the E2β addition. Similarly, capsaicin stimulation in a Ca^{2+}-free media with 10 mM BAPTA eliminated $[Ca^{2+}]_i$ fluxes.

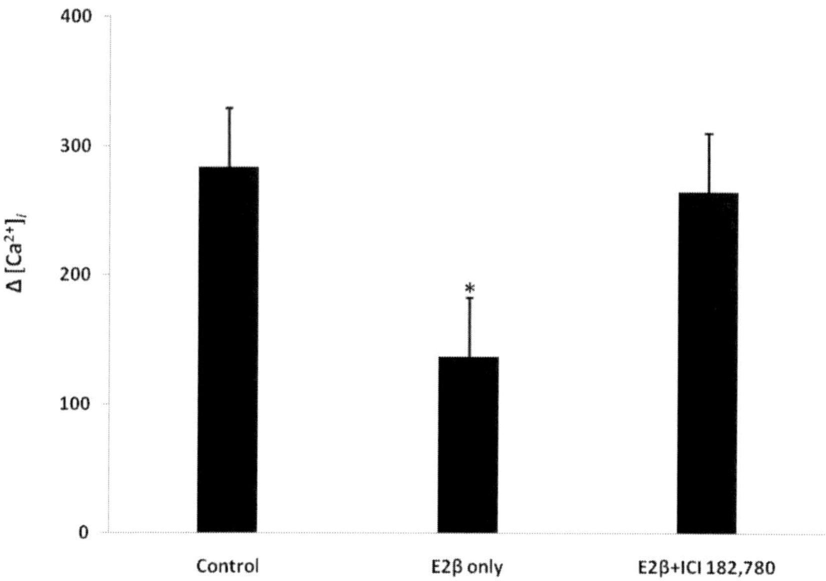

Figure 7.3. Summary data of control, 17β-estradiol (E2β), and E2β + ICI 182,780 effects on capsaicin-induced $[Ca^{2+}]_i$ fluxes change in DRG neurons. The amplitudes of $\Delta [Ca^{2+}]_i$ changes were determined by subtracting the $[Ca^{2+}]_i$ fluxes from the basal $[Ca^{2+}]_i$ levels during capsaicin stimulation. Addition 17β-estradiol (E2β, 100 nM) significantly decreased $[Ca^{2+}]_i$ response to capsaicin while estrogen receptor antagonist ICI 182,780 (1 μM) blocked E2β effect. Values are expressed as mean ± SEM $P<0.05$, n=10 per group. * indicate significant difference from control, $P < 0.05$.

To identify the role of ER subtype, both ERα and ERβ, mediated with E2β modulation of capsaicin-induced $[Ca^{2+}]_i$ transients, we tested E2β attenuation of $[Ca^{2+}]_i$ responses using the DRG neurons from Wt, ERαKO and ERβKO mice. We found the similarity of E2β effect in ERβKO mouse DRG neurons to that observed in Wt mouse. In contrast, ERαKO mouse show that E2β did not inhibit capsaicin-induced $[Ca^{2+}]_i$ transients, indicating that it depends on ERα 17α-estradiol had no effect on Wt, ERαKO, or ERβKO mouse. Our data indicated that DRG neurons in culture can be used to study the cellular response to a putative nociceptive signal, and 17β-estradiol attenuates the capsaicin-induced $[Ca^{2+}]_i$ responses and interferes with the membrane-associated ERα.

Peripheral sensitization can develop in response to sustain stimulation, inflammation, and nerve injury. Visceral pain is different from cutaneous pain based on clinical, neurophysiological, and pharmacological characteristics

(Chang and Heitkemper 2002). In the contest to visceral pain, the TRPV1 receptor is a sensory neuron-specific cation channel which belongs to the transient receptor potential subfamily 1 and plays an important role in transporting thermal and inflammatory pain signals. TRPV1 receptors are distributed in peripheral sensory nerve endings and are involved in the transduction of different stimuli in sensory neurons. TRPV1 functions as molecular integrator of painful chemical and physical stimuli (noxious heat (>43ºC) and low pH). Various inflammatory mediators such as prostaglandin E2 (PGE2) and bradykinin potentiate TRPV1. The potentiating of TRPV1 activity can be quantified by measuring the differences of capsaicin-induced Ca2+ concentration changes before and after receptor activation (Petruska et al. 2000). Significantly, a subset of DRG neurons respond to both capsaicin and ATP (Canti et al. 1999) indicating that there may be cross-activation of these receptors that may underlie the sensitization of visceral nociceptors. Although large numbers of clinical and animal studies have indicated that there are sex and estrous cycle differences in pain perception of various pain models (Fillingim et al. 1997; Bradshaw et al. 2000; Craft et al. 2004; Cook and Nickerson, 2005; Gazerani et al. 2005), it remains unclear whether sex and estrous cycle differences in capsaicin-induced acute pain also occur in mice. It is well known and documented that capsaicin evokes a subset of mammalian sensory neurons. This results from activation of a ligand-gated nonselective cation channel with subsequent membrane depolarization and action potential generation (Bevan and Szolcsanyi 1990; Marsh et al. 1987; Oh et al. 1996). Indeed, such a channel, TRPV1, has been cloned (Caterina et al. 1997) and found to be expressed in various types of sensory neurons (Caterinal et al. 1997; Helliwell et al. 1998; Tominaga et al. 1998). This study showed that capsaicin-induced $[Ca^{2+}]_i$ transients evoked in small- and medium-size DRG neurons. The response was inhibited by capsazepine (300 nM), a antagonist of the TRPV1, and was rely on the extracellular $[Ca^{2+}]_i$ transients. These data demonstrate the mouse DRG neurons in culture retain the same responses to a rapid application of E2β as mouse cultured DRG, providing us with an additional tool of ER 'knock-outs' for studying the effects of E2β. 17β-estradiol acts through an ERα in modulating the TRPV1 receptor-mediated $[Ca^{2+}]_i$ response in DRG, since its effect was eliminated in ERαKO mouse and retained in ERβKO. The present results demonstrate an important nonreproductive role of ERα in modulating capsaicin-induced Ca^{2+} signaling at the level of the primary afferent neuron, thereby modulating the sensitivity to painful stimuli in the periphery. Furthermore, E2β plays a crucial role in the sex steroids difference in capsaicin-induced nociception in mouse. These findings are consistent with our previous our data that E2β potentiates the TRPV1-mediated responses in mouse DRG neurons. The mechanism underlying the effect of E2β on the TRPV1-mediated nociceptive response needs further investigation. A better understanding of how E2β potentiates capsaicin-induced nociception may offer a new clinical therapeutic strategy for pain management.

Role of TRPV1 and P2X2/3 Receptors in Visceral Nociception Mediated by ERα in DRG Neurons

Our previous studies showed DRG neurons innervating viscera are about 5-10%. A corollary of that hypothesis is that cutaneous pain may show different action of pain modulation compared with visceral pain. Even though there are no changes in cutaneous modulation of pain, pathologically visceral modulation of pain such as inflammation and IBS is more prevalent in women. This experiment is designed to compare the pharmacology of retrogradely labeled visceral DRG neurons with retrogradely labeled cutaneous DRG neurons. Within the context of our hypothesis, nociceptive responses by E2 modulation depend on the kinds of pain, its durations. To find mechanism of viscero/visceral hyperalgesia between organs including viscero/visceral-somatic convergent neurons, retrograde labeling was used to demonstrate cultured DRG neurons receiving sensory signaling input from different visceral organs such as colon and uterus. We inject fluorogold (FG) to colon and tetramethylrhodamine (TMR) to uterus into the muscle wall by abdominal incision and somatic afferent neurons (Alexa Fluor 647) by subcutaneous injection into mouse hind paw. Both uterine and colonic afferents were shown in DRG neurons. Retrogradely labeled visceral DRG cells that project to the colon or uterus were co-localized in the same DRG neuron, suggesting a subpopulation of DRG neurons that innervate both colon and uterus. These DRG neurons innervating both colon and uterus represent a new group of dichotomizing sensory afferents. In addition, E2 (100 nM) by itself had no effect on basal $[Ca^{2+}]i$, but the ATP-induced $[Ca^{2+}]i$ flux was decreased by this hormone. After the initial ATP response, incubation with E2 for five minute inhibited ATP-induced $[Ca^{2+}]i$ transient. On the other hand, retrogradely labeled cutaneous DRG neurons injecting to hind paw were shown in the DRG cells. These neurons did not block ATP-induced $[Ca^{2+}]_i$ and showed low amplitudes of E2 effects on ATP-induced $[Ca^{2+}]_i$ response.

The effect of E2 modulation of P2X2/3 and TRPV1 receptors mediated $[Ca^{2+}]_i$ response in both retrogradely labeled visceral and cutaneous DRG neurons DRG neurons innervating viscera demonstrated greater amplitudes of E2 effects on ATP-induced $[Ca^{2+}]_i$ response suggesting that neurons innervating visceral organs may express and regulate ER differently. ER is more tightly coupled to P2X2/3 and TRPV1. To identify of E2 modulation of calcium responses from retrogradely labeled visceral and somatic neurons, we also used α, β-meATP, a specific agonist of P2X2/3, to confirm the observations presented with ATP. Both P2X2/3 and P2X3 receptors have similar properties and seem to be a target for estradiol. Moreover, TRPV1 receptors can be activated by capsaicin and regulated by inflammatory mediators including PGE2 and bradykinin (Dray 2008), whose effects are mediated through an increase of $[Ca^{2+}]_i$ in mouse DRG neurons. The E2 had no effect of calcium changes by itself, but E2 (100 nM) showed low intensity of capsaicin-induced $[Ca^{2+}]_i$ transients. The superfusion with capsaicin (100 nM) induced $[Ca^{2+}]_i$ increases, but this effect was diminished by E2. There was statistically significant difference the effect of TRPV1 in wild type mice. However, there are no effect and smaller E2 effect on α, β-meATP/capsaicin-induced $[Ca^{2+}]_i$ responses in retrogradely labeled somatic DRG neurons compared with visceral DRG neurons. These results suggest that the E2 effects on TRPV1 seemed to be one of the signaling pathways for E2-mediated changes of TRPV1 activity and the pain perception of visceral afferents.

The role of ERα/ERβ in E2 modulation on α, β-meATP- and capsaicin-induced $[Ca^{2+}]_i$ transients in retrogradely labeled visceral and cutaneous mouse DRG neurons. To verify the role of ERα and ERβ in the potentially different response from visceral and somatic DRG neurons, visceral DRG neurons retrogradely labeled with Fluorogold for colonic afferents and TMR for uterine afferents were stimulated with either α,β-meATP or capsaicin and compared to differences from retrogradely labeled somatic DRG neurons in knock-out mice. The E2 effects in ERβKO mouse DRG neurons show similar to wild type mice. However, in ERαKO mice there are no E2 effects on α, β-meATP-induced $[Ca^{2+}]_i$ fluxes. 17α-Estradiol, a different isomer of 17β-estradiol, had no effect on Wt, ERαKO or ERβKO mice. We also demonstrated capsaicin-induced $[Ca^{2+}]_i$ changes in knock-out mice to find the examination presented with capsaicin in wild type mice. We also found the similarity of E2 effects in ERβKO to that presented in wild type mice, but E2 didn't show any differences in ERαKO mice on capsaicin-induced $[Ca^{2+}]_i$ fluxes. Our study used a combined approach to decide that primary cultured DRG neurons can be used to research the cellular reaction to a nociceptive α,β-meATP-sensitive P2X2/3 and capsaicin-sensitive TRPV1 receptors. In retrogradely labeled somatic DRG neurons, however E2 didn't inhibit and show low intensity on α, β-meATP/capsaicin-induced $[Ca^{2+}]_i$ fluxes. Our data suggest that sensory DRG neurons innervating viscera demonstrate greater amplitudes of E2 effects on the α, β-meATP/capsaicin-induced $[Ca^{2+}]_i$ fluxes and E2 interfere with the membrane-associated ERα in viscerally-specific neurons.

Comparison of the effects of E2 on PGE2 potentiation of TRPV1-mediated calcium response in retrogradely labeled visceral and cutaneous DRG neurons from Wt, ERαKO, and ERβKO mice. The action of E2 is important to determine the physiological properties of ERs expressed in visceral neurons and which ER mediates E2 effects in visceral compared with somatic DRG neurons (Figure 7.4).

In addition, methodologically it is very difficult to study receptor activation on the neuritis of DRG neurons. An underlying assumption of these studies is that receptors located on peripheral terminals of colonic primary afferent neurons have the same functional properties as those expressed on the soma of DRG neurons (Gold 1996). Hence in vitro DRG neurons are the best model for the proposed experiments. It is hypothesized that ERs on colonic primary afferent neurons may have different functional properties compared with those expressed on somatic afferent neurons. The potentiating of TRPV1 is considered to be important in pain process from inflammation. Moreover, E2 is more likely to magnify higher intensities of PGE2-mediated TRPV1 activation in retrogradely labeled visceral DRG neurons than in somatic DRG neurons. To confirm whether ERα or ERβ play an important role in E2 pretreatment before the addition of PGE2 (100 nM) on capsaicin-induced calcium responses, retrogradely labeled DRG neurons from Wt, ERαKO, and ERβKO mice were used. In retrogradely labeled visceral DRG neurons, after pretreatment with PGE2, the E2 mediated $[Ca^{2+}]_i$ transients by capsaicin was elevated from a control condition (data not shown).

This study suggested that capsaicin-induced $[Ca^{2+}]$i transients were enhanced after the PGE2 pretreatment by almost 2~3 fold. However, the E2 by itself had no effect on basal $[Ca^{2+}]_i$, but E2 (100 nM) in the presence of inflammatory mediator, PGE2, attenuated the intensities of capsaicin-induced $[Ca^{2+}]_i$ transients in wild. Especially, we tested the role of ERβ in the context of the influence of PGE2-mediated capsaicin-induced $[Ca^{2+}]_i$ fluxes.

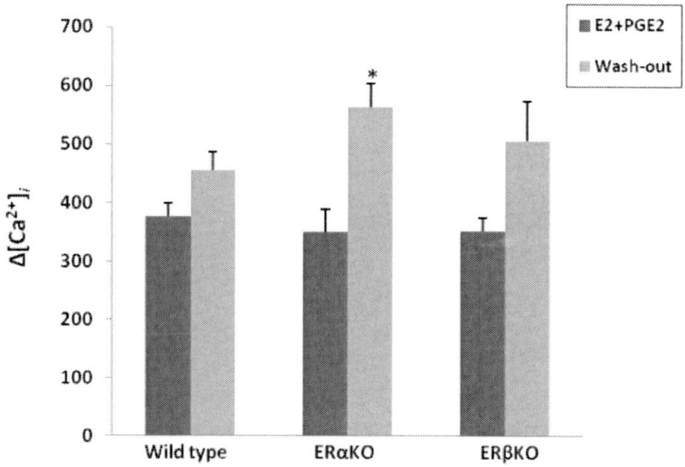

a

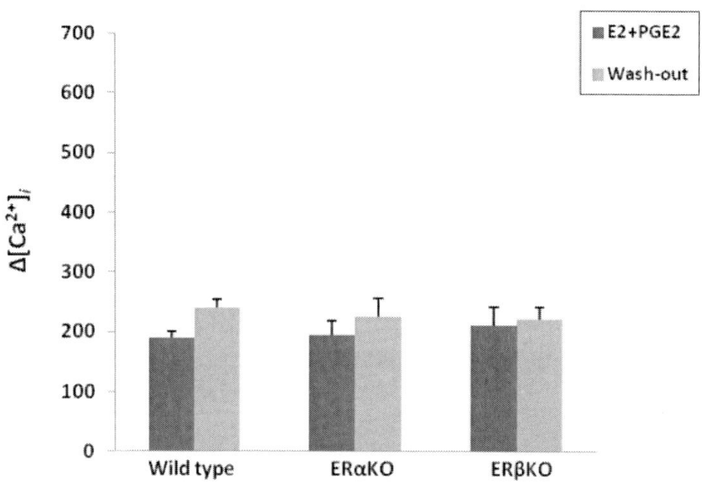

b

Figure 7.4. Summary of PGE2 pontentiation of capsaicin-induced $[Ca^{2+}]_i$ transients of control and the presence of E2 in visceral and somatic DRG neurons from wild type, ERαKO, and ERβKO mice. Summary data represented on the right bar graphs. E2 significantly decreased $[Ca^{2+}]_i$ response to (a) PGE2 potentiated capsaicin in ERαKO mice but somatic DRG neurons had no statistically significant E2 effect on (b) PGE2 potentiated capsaicin and there are low intensities calcium changes compared visceral DRG neurons. Values are expressed as mean ± SEM. * indicate statistically significant difference from control, $P < 0.05$.

The effect of PGE2 after E2 pretreatment was similar in ERβKO mouse DRG neurons to that observed in Wt mice but, E2 did not block capsaicin-induced $[Ca^{2+}]_i$ in DRG neurons from ERαKO mice suggesting that its diminution depends on ERα. However E2 didn't work on capsaicin-induced $[Ca^{2+}]_i$ responses in the retrogradely labeled somatic DRG neurons.

Our data suggest that visceral DRG neurons show higher intensities of E2 effects on PGE2-mediated capsaicin-induced $[Ca^{2+}]_i$ fluxes and E2 interfere with the membrane-associated ERα in viscerally-specific neurons. PGE2 could potentiate the response of the TRPV1 and E2 effects on TRPV1 under pathological conditions such as inflammation might be one of the pain signaling pathways. This data confirmed that the role of ERα and not ERβ in the E2 modulates PGE2-mediated TRPV1 activation in visceral DRG neurons. These present situation can reflect patients suffering from pathological abdominal pain in clinical studies for many functional disorders. Visceral hyperalgesia is considered to be an important signaling pathways of functional pain syndromes associated with patients of IBS, PBS, and CPP. The mechanisms of viscero-visceral cross-sensitization play an important role in the demonstration of visceral pain syndromes affecting different organs often coexist. Although it is usually understood that each primary sensory neuron is a single channel, several studies have demonstrated that DRG neurons can innervate both visceral and somatic organs. This study using retrograde labeling from uterus and colon gave important challenges that the same sensory neuron can innervate both reproductive and gastrointestinal organs. These dichotomized fibers provide a novel mechanism for sensitization of one internal organ by another. Our study show that DRG neurons that innervate both colon and uterus in short-term culture express capsaicin-sensitive TRPV1 receptors and ATP-sensitive P2X3/α, β-meATP-sensitive P2X2/3 receptors which mediate the response to putative nociceptive signals. Our findings suggest that sensory information to the sensory neurons may initiate in different viscera. ER agonists mimic activation of these receptors in vivo. Moreover, these neurons can be a good model of endogenous signals. Many literatures suggest that E2 modulation of nociceptive pain processing in functional pain disorders. Within our hypothesis, E2 modulation depends on pain types, durations, and other anti-nociceptive signaling pathways. Thus, E2 modulates short-cultured sensory DRG neurons to capsaicin and ATP/α, β-meATP, suggesting that visceral nociceptive neurons are modulated by E2, which can manifest clinical findings, animal sex-differences associated with visceral hyperalgesia, and a potential target for mediating nociception. In addition, E2 modulation of viscero-visceral cross sensitization appear in DRG neurons and P2X3/P2X2/3 and TRPV1 receptors in retrogradely labeled visceral DRG neurons attenuated ATP/α, β-meATP/capsaicin-induced $[Ca^{2+}]_i$ fluxes, but retrogradely labeled somatic DRG neurons didn't inhibit $[Ca^{2+}]_i$ responses, suggesting that nociceptive signals modulate peripherally visceral pain sensitization in vitro.

Nociceptive mechanisms including the functional pain syndromes are complicated by co-morbid disorders. Visceral nociception and nociceptor sensitization appear to be regulated by ATP/capsaicin. The medium (diameter<40 microns) and small (diameter <25 microns) DRG neurons in short-term culture respond to ATP/capsaicin and were estrogen-sensitive, indicating that there may be cross-activation of these receptors that may underlie the pain perception of visceral nociceptors. Although large numbers of clinical and animal studies have indicated that there are sex and estrous cycle differences in pain perception of various pain models, it remains unclear whether sex and estrous cycle differences in ATP/capsaicin-induced acute pain also occur in mice. Furthermore, the PGE2 is synthesized and released in response to damaged tissues, contributes to hyperalgesia, and is involved in the acute and chronic inflammatory reactions. The E2 is anti-nociceptive and decrease capsaicin-induced $[Ca^{2+}]_i$ responses without PGE2 present.

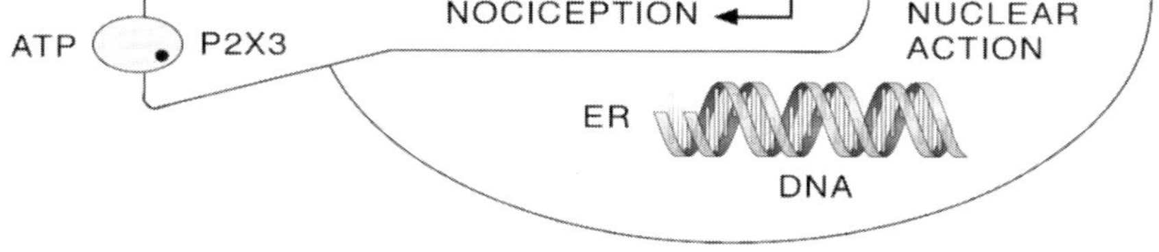

Figure 7.5. Proposed mechanism of 17-βestradiol (E2) effect on ATP-induced $[Ca^{2+}]_i$ signaling in primary sensory neurons. ATP released by tissue damage acts on P2X3 receptor resulting in activation of the L-type voltage-gated calcium channel (L-VGCC). ERα modulates ATP-induced P2X3- mediated as well as capsaicin-induced TRPV1-mediated $[Ca^{2+}]_i$ increases in DRGs.

In our previous studies showed that PGE2 enhanced the Ca^{2+} responses induced by ATP and capsaicin. This data indicated that the sensitizing actions of PGE2 on retrogradely labeled visceral DRG neurons are mediated through the pain signaling pathway such as cAMP/PKA. Within the context of our hypothesis visceral nociception and nociceptor sensitization appear to be regulated by purinergic P2X3 and vanilloid TRPV1 receptors and 17β-estradiol modulates DRG neurons response to ATP (P2X3 agonist) and capsaicin (TRPV1 agonist), suggesting that visceral afferent nociceptors are modulated by estrogen in the DRG. Based on our data, we proposed that E2 can gate the primary afferent response to increase or decrease nociception (Figure 7.5).

References

Bevan S and Szolcsanyi J. Sensory neuron-specific actions of capsaicin: mechanisms and applications. *Trends Pharmacol Sci.*1990, 11:330-333.

Beyak, M.J. and S. Vanner, Inflammation-induced hyperexcitability of nociceptive gastrointestinal DRG neurones: the role of voltage-gated ion channels. *Neurogastroenterol Motil,* 2005. 17(2): p. 175-186.

Bradshaw H, Miller J, Ling Q, Malsnee K, and Ruda MA. Sex differences and phases of the estrous cycle alter the response of spinal cord dynorphin neurons to peripheral inflammation and hyperalgesia. *Pain*, 2000, 85:93-99.

Canti C, Page KM, Stephens GJ, Dolphin AC. Identification of residues in the N terminus of alpha1B critical for inhibition of the voltage-dependent calcium channel by G beta gamma. *J Neurosci.,* 1999, 19(16):6855-6864.

Caterina MJ, Leffler A, Malmberg AB, Martin WJ, Trafton J, Petersen-Zeitz KR, Koltzenburg M, Basbaum AI, Julius D. Impaired nociception and pain sensation in mice lacking the capsaicin receptor. *Science,* 2000. 288:306-313.

Caterina MJ, Schumacher MA, Tominaga M, Rosen TA, Levine JD, Julius D (1997). The capsaicin receptor: a heat-activated ion channel in the pain pathway. *Nature,* 1997, 389:816-824.

Chaban VV, McRoberts JA, Ennes HS, Mayer EA. Nitric oxide synthase inhibitors enhance mechanosensitive Ca^{2+} influx in cultured dorsal root ganglion neurons. *Brain Res.* 2001, 903(1-2):74-85.

Chaban V. Peripheral sensitization of sensory neurons. *Ethn Dis.,* 2010, 20:S1-3-6.

Chang L, Heitkemper MM. Gender differences in irritable bowel syndrome. *Gastroenterology,* 2001, 123(5):1686-1701.

Cook CD and Nickerson MD. Nociceptive sensitivity and opioid antinociception and antihyperalgesia in Freund's adjuvant-induced arthritic male and female rats. *J Pharmacol Exp Ther.,* 2005, 313:449-459.

Craft RM, Mogil JS, and Aloisi AM. Sex differences in pain and analgesia: the role of gonadal hormones. *Eur J Pain.* 2004, 8:397-411.

Dai, Y., et al. Contribution of sensitized P2X receptors in inflamed tissue to the mechanical hypersensitivity revealed by phosphorylated ERK in DRG neurons. *Pain,* 2004. 108(3): p. 258-66.

Davis JB, Gray J, Gunthorpe MJ, Hatcher JP, Davey PT, Overend P, Harries MH, Latcham J, Clapham C, Atkinson K, Hughes SA, Rance K, Grau E, Harper AJ, Pugh PL, Rogers DC, Bingham S, Randall A, Sheardown SA Vanilloid receptor-1 is essential for inflammatory thermal hyperalgesia. *Nature,* 2000, 405(6783):183-187.

Dray A. Neuropathic pain: emerging treatments. *British J* 2008. Anesthesia 101(1): 48-58.

Eun SY, Jung SJ, Park YK, Kwak J, Kim SJ, Kim J. Effect of capsaicin on Ca^{2+} release from the intracellular Ca^{2+} stores in the dorsal root ganglion cells of adult rats. *Biochem Biophys Res Commun,* 2001, 285(5):1114-1120.

Fillingim RB, Maixner W, Girdler SS, Light KC, Harris MB, Sheps DS, and Mason GA. Ischemic but not thermal pain sensitivity varies across the menstrual cycle. *Psychosom Med,* 1997, 59:512-520.

Gazerani P, Andersen OK, and Arendt-Nielsen L. A human experimental capsaicin model for trigeminal sensitization. Gender-specific differences. *Pain,* 2005, 118:155-163.

Gold MS, Dastmalchi S, Levine JD. Co-expressed of nociceptor properties in dorsal root ganglion neurons from the adult rat in vitro. *Neuroscience* 1996. 71(1): 265-275.

Helliwell RJ, Mclatchie LM, Clarke M, Winter J, Beven S, Mcintyre P. Capsaicin sensitivity is associated with the expression of the vanilloid (capsaicin) receptor (VR1) mRNA in adult rat sensory ganglia. *Neurosci Lett.*, 2008, 250:177-180.

Jankowski, M.P. and H.R. Koerber, *Neurotrophic Factors and Nociceptor Sensitization.* 2010.

Koshimizu, TA, Van Goor F, Tomić M, Wong AO, Tanoue A, Tsujimoto G, Stojikovic. S., Characterization of calcium signaling by purinergic receptor-channels expressed in excitable cells. *Mol Pharmacol.*, 2000, 58(5):936-945.

Li, J., et al. Experimental colitis modulates the functional properties of NMDA receptors in dorsal root ganglia neurons. *Am J Physiol Gastrointest Liver Physiol*, 2006. 291(2): p. G219-28.

Marsh SJ, Stansfeld CE, Brown DA, Davey R, Mccarthy D. The mechanism of action of capsaicin on sensory C-type neurons and their axons in vitro. *Neuroscience,* 1987, 23:275-289.

Negri, L., et al. Impaired nociception and inflammatory pain sensation in mice lacking the prokineticin receptor PKR1: focus on interaction between PKR1 and the capsaicin receptor TRPV1 in pain behavior. *J Neurosci,* 2006. 26(25): p. 6716-27.

Oh U, Hwang SW, Kim D. Capsaicin activates a nonselective cation channel in cultured neonatal rat dorsal root ganglion neurons. *J Neurosci.* 1996, 16:1659-1667.

Petruska JC, Napaporn J, Johnson RD, Gu JG, Cooper BY. Subclassified acutely dissociated cells of rat DRG: histochemistry and patterns of capsaicin-, proton-, and ATP-activated currents. *J Neurophysiol.*. 2000 84(5):2365-2379.

Tominaga M, Caterina MJ, Malmberg AB, Rosen TA, Gilbert H, Skinner K, Raumann BE, Basbaum AI, Julium D. The cloned capsaicin receptor integrates multiple pain-producing stimuli. *Neuron,* 1998, 21:531-543.

Waxman SG, Cummins TR, Dib-Hajj SD, Black JA. Voltage-gated sodium channels and the molecular pathogenesis of pain: a review. *J Rehabil Res Dev,* 2000, 37, 5517– 5528.

Xu, G.Y. and L.Y. Huang, Peripheral inflammation sensitizes P2X receptor-mediated responses in rat dorsal root ganglion neurons. *J Neurosci*, 2002. 22(1): p. 93-102.

Future Perspectives

The accumulation of nociceptive diseases that limit normal body functions is a major risk factor for disability, and visceral pain is one of the most prevalent human health problem. Many pain-associated neurodegenerative diseases are accompanied by the concomitant decline in cognitive and motor performance. Cells of the affected neuronal tissues may interact in cell-to-cell manner messages through the transfer of hormones, cytokines, and autacoids that are released or modified in such pathological conditions. The complex interplay and balance between these diverse mediators, genetic background, and environmental factors may ultimately determine the outcome of nociceptive progression. Primary afferent neurons (otherwise known as sensory neurons), carry nerve impulses from receptors of cutaneous and visceral sense organs for processing within the central nervous system.

Clinical studies suggest the comorbidity of functional pain syndromes such as Irritable Bowel Syndrome (IBS), Painful Bladder Syndrome (PBS), and Chronic Pelvic Pain (CPP). Persistent, episodic, or chronic visceral pain is more prevalent in females, thus defining the site(s) and mechanisms of modulation of visceral nociception is an important step in understanding the gender differences in pain perception and in designing appropriate therapies. Recent studies from our laboratory and others about function of estrogen receptors (ER) in DRG neurons strongly suggest that 17β-estradiol (E2) modulates visceral pain processing peripherally (Chaban 2013). E2 (both short-term and long-term exposure) significantly decreased the nociceptive signaling in viscerally-labeled DRG neurons suggesting that estradiol may affect nociception peripherally. Pain in general and specifically pelvic pain is subjective feeling and thus difficult to standardize and parameterize in a mathematical fashion for scientific analysis. Often, the etiology of visceral pain is not clear, as there are many symptoms of the reproductive system, gastrointestinal and urinary tracts, musculoskeletal, neurological and psychological systems that often co-occur in the same patient. Viscero-somatic and viscero-viseral hyperalgesia and allodynia result in the spread of a perception of pain from an initial site to adjacent areas (Malykhina 2007). The variation of pain symptoms and pain perception, and behavioral responses to pain in these patients, is poorly understood. The treating clinician is often tempted to take a unidimensional approach and focus on one organ system and ignore the psychological and behavioral manifestations of the chronic pain.

There is often no clear relationship between the severity of the chronic pelvic pain and pathology in the pelvic viscera, including the reproductive tract (ovaries and uterus), urinary bladder, and colon. Studies of the sympathetic nervous system in individuals with CPP associated with gynecological diseases, painful bladder syndrome/interstitial cystitis (IC) and functional bowel disorders such as irritable bowel syndrome (IBS), suggest a model in which alteration in the central stress circuits in predisposed individuals may be triggered by and then maintain the pain and pathophysiological changes in the viscera (Mayer 2011). CPP patients have significantly more depression, psychological and somatic complains and more often give a history of physical, sexual or emotional abuse, or trauma. Chronic pain adversely affects mood, social, and professional life and general well-being. These quality of life issues can affect the severity of pain, degree of impairment resulting from a painful condition and success of pain treatment modalities in alleviating pain. Because of the inherent subjectivity of pain, there is a wide disparity among individuals in the way that they experience the pain generated by what seem to be similar stimuli. There is also a tension between the subjectivity of the patient's pain experience and the common insistence of the clinician upon objective findings that are proportionate with the patient's complaints to enable to distinguish between exaggerated pain reports.

In the United States, pain accounts for nearly 20% of all primary health care visits. For the last couple of decades, medical literature has carefully documented the undertreatment of all types of pain by physicians. During this period, the phenomenon of undertreated pain received almost no attention from the medical community (Barsky et al. 2005). There are two essential components of pain: discriminative and affective. The discriminative component includes the ability to identify the stimulus as originating from somatic or visceral tissue, determine some of the physical properties of the stimulus, and localize it in space, time, and along a continuum of intensities. The affective component is the experience which motivates escape, avoidance, and protective behavior. All of these components of pain must be considered in any discussion of the neurophysiological basis of pain. A consideration of pain mechanisms must also include the neural systems modulating pain, for it is well known that pain can be profoundly influenced by other somatic stimuli and by attentional, emotional, and cognitive factors. History and physical examinations are crucial in evaluating a suffering patient and must address all of the possible systems potentially involved in chronic pelvic pain, not just the reproductive system. Assessing the impact of the pain on various domains of a patient's existence has become an important focus in clinical management. Pain is a complex and individual experience that is often difficult for patients to fully describe using a conventional clinical assessment. The health-related quality of life encompasses those aspects of health and well-being valued by patients, specifically, their physical, emotional, and cognitive function, and their ability to participate in meaningful activities within their family, workplace, and community. There is concern that not enough emphasis is placed on clinical face validity (i.e., issues which are important to patients and reflect their experiences). A balance between biomedical, organ-oriented, and cognitive interpersonal approaches is most appropriate at this truly psychosomatic interface. In view of the iatrogenic component in the maintenance of functional somatic syndromes, doctor-centered interventions and close observation of the doctor-patient relationship are of particular importance.

Pelvic pain affects up to 25% of women at some time in their lives (about a billion worldwide) and can result in dysmenorrhea, dyspareunia, menstrual irregularities, back pain, gastrointestinal and genitourinary symptoms, and reduced fecundity. The incidents of persistent visceral pain associated with functional disorders such as IBS, CPP, PBS and others is 2-3 times higher in women than in men suggesting E2 modulation. A large body of literature supports the idea that estrogen modulates nociceptive responses in pelvic pain syndromes; however, whether this hormone is pro- or anti-nociceptive remains unresolved. The concept that brain and other visceral systems (i.e., gastrointestinal and genitourinary) are closely connected and that this interaction plays an important role in certain feeling states especially in clinical presentations of chronic viscerally-associated nociceptive disorders is widely accepted in scientific and clinical communities (Mayer 2011). In women, pain symptoms and nociceptive thresholds vary with reproductive cycle, and our data strongly suggest the role of estrogen receptors in the modulation of nociceptive signaling (Chaban 2012). Moreover, our data that estrogen can gate the primary afferent response to modulate nociception supports the idea of the involvement of the peripheral central system in the etiology of a wide range of functional and inflammatory gastrointestinal diseases and may potentially lead to new interventions and therapies. The DRG is an important site of visceral afferent convergence and cross-sensitization.

Nociceptive responses are highly complex, involving a vast array of messenger molecules interacting with enzymes and receptors of virtually every class, directing recruitment of many types of cells to recover the healthy state. Indeed, a balance between the messengers with the inherent redundancy of the different body systems makes therapeutic intervention a considerable challenge. The localization of ER in DRG neurons and the attenuation of ATP/capsaicin- induce $[Ca^{2+}]_i$ strongly suggests that E2 modulates visceral pain processing peripherally. 17-β estradiol (E2), the most common form of estrogen, acts on functional properties of P2X3 and TRPV1 receptors in DRG neurons. Experimental long-term (chronic) exposure to E2 on sensory neurons can mimic the temporal pattern of circulating E2 levels in cycling female rodents, which is equivalent to an E2 primal action on animal reproductive behavior. Cells of the affected tissues may interact in a cell-to-cell manner messages through the transfer of hormones, cytokines, and autacoids such as histamine, serotonin, kinins and prostaglandins that are released in pathological processes. The complex interplay and balance between these diverse mediators, ageing, genetic background, and environmental factors may ultimately determine the outcome of progression of chronic nociception. On a molecular level, these responses are highly complex, involving a vast array of messenger molecules interacting with enzymes and receptors of virtually every class, directing recruitment of many types of cells to recover the healthy state. Indeed, a balance between the messengers with the inherent redundancy of the different body systems makes therapeutic intervention a considerable challenge. The impact on society of a successful translation of a basic or clinical observation into new therapies is substantial, taking into consideration the rapid growth of scientific knowledge. Today, understanding and meeting public concerns are as important for the investigator as performing research studies. Sex steroid hormones are thought as indispensable cornerstones of the normal development and function, but it appears that nobody region, no neuronal circuit, and virtually no cell is unaffected by them. Estrogen can affect nociception and many other systems thus, increasing awareness toward hormones appears to be obligatory. New data regarding our understanding of the mechanisms of estrogen modulation of visceral pain will hopefully lead to the development of effective gender-specific therapies for functional disorders.

In most nociceptive disease affecting visceral organs, there is a striking gender-differences in their etiology. More than a decade ago, the Unites States Institute of Medicine report, "Exploring the Biological Contribution to Human Health," confirmed that differences between the sexes exist in the prevalence and severity of a broad range of diseases, disorders and conditions. In calling for greater focus on gender-based biomedical research, the IOM report identified barriers to the achievement of knowledge about gender differences, including ethical, financial, sociological and scientific factors. In the United States, pain accounts for nearly 20% of all primary health care visits. Studies have shown that at least one-third of patients with visceral pain also suffer from depression, and it affects more women than men. Projects described in this book address a crucial question in women's health and in visceral nociception in particular. Reaching further, this project is a liaison between the basic science work and the clinical aspects that are addressed through other disciplines such as anesthesiology (pain management), gastroenterology and gynecology. The author aims to help qualified professionals in clinical research methodologies, biostatistics, clinical trials, collaborative science, and research conduct, to provide a unique understanding of the numerous issues in pain research, as well as to describe potentially new therapies with a core emphasis on new mechanisms. The author is well poised to take advantage of his current basic scientific and clinical interests within this area, to contribute substantial information towards the treatment of gender-based pelvic pain disorders.

As with all new stories, the "unusual" in science and medicine gets the attention of the general public. With immediate access to health information through the internet, many patients have differences of opinion regarding certain topics compared to their provider. In that case we need to convey to patients and the general public through currently available sources (publications, media) that we understand the constant challenges of searching for the most effective therapies.

We need to convey the message that new research will drive progress. Translational science has a major, immediate impact on future therapies and improvement on quality of life for patients. Before leaving readers to find their own path into this intriguing field of visceral pain, let me make some conclusions. The present day therapies useful in treatment of nociceptive diseases arose, for the most part, without good insight into the nature of disease, so, readers: start your own exploration!

References

Barsky, A.J. et al. Somatization increases medical utilization and costs independent of psychiatric and medical comorbidity. *Arch Gen Psychiatry* 2005. 62(8): p. 903-10.

Chaban, V., et al. Estradiol attenuates the adenosine triphosphate-induced increase of intracellular calcium through group II metabotropic glutamate receptors in rat dorsal root ganglion neurons. *J Neurosci Res*, 2011. 89(11): p. 1707-10.

Chaban, V. Estrogen and Visceral Nociception at the Level of Primary Sensory Neurons. *Pain Res Treat*, 2012.

Chaban V. Primary Afferent Nociceptors and Visceral Pain, Endometriosis - Basic Concepts and Current Research Trends ISBN:978-953-51-0524-4, *InTech*, 2012, p. 367-381Chaban V.

Chaban V. Estrogen modulation of visceral nociceptors. *Current Trends in Neurology* 2013. 7: p. 51- 54.

Chaban V. Chronic pelvic pain: focus on etiology and modulation. Int. J Res in Nursing, 2014. 5(1): p. 1-2.

Malykhina, A.P. Neural mechanisms of pelvic organ cross-sensitization. *Neuroscience,* 2007. 149(3): p. 660-72.

Mayer E. Gut feelings: the emerging biology of gut- brain communication. *Nat Rev Neurosci* 2011. 12(8): p. 453- 466.

Meltzak R. Pain and the Neuromatrix in the Brain, 2001. *J Dent Educ* 65(12): p.1378–82.

Index

A

B

C

D

E

F

G

H

I

J

K

L

M

N

O

P

Q

R

S

T